D0241010

*To anyone who is willing to take that
first step to leading a healthier life*

CONTENTS

WELLBEING

SIMPLE BUT EFFECTIVE TIPS TO HELP YOU STAY ON TRACK

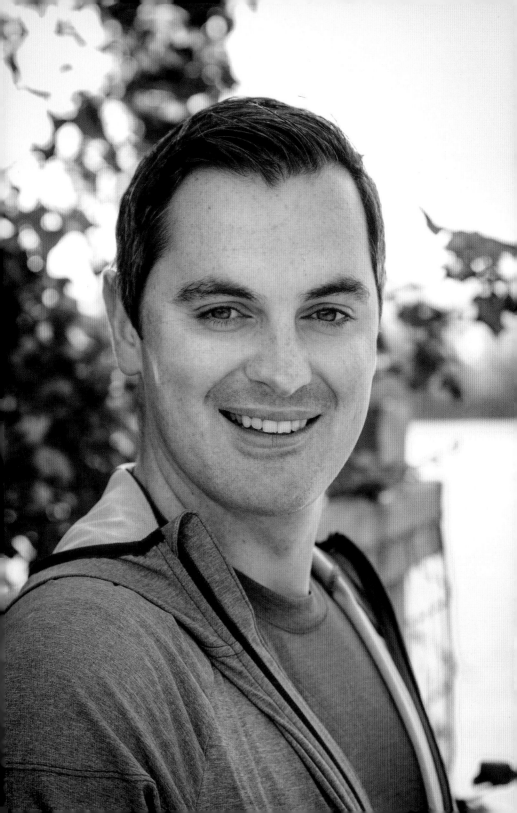

INTRODUCTION

Just like in the rest of the Western world, in Ireland there is a growing divide in the population between the fit and unfit, the healthy and unhealthy, the average and overweight. At one extreme, there is a category of health-conscious people who are very focused on eating nutritiously and exercising regularly. And at the other, there are a lot of people making poor choices, who eat high-sugar, highly processed foods and take little exercise. And in the middle? Those who muddle through on a diet of the good and not-so-great, who try to fit a bit of regular movement into their lives but occasionally succumb to their couch-potato tendencies, who go through phases of being 'good' and phases of life making it difficult to stick with the healthier-living intentions.

In nearly 20 years as a personal trainer, I have seen it all. Apart from those who are already health-conscious, I have worked extensively with the other two groups – people who thought there was no hope of changing their lives and also those who doubted their ability to make the best choices on an ongoing basis. I hope this book will be of particular benefit to these two groups – those who have woken up to the importance of taking their lifestyle in hand, and those who already know a lot of the things they need to do to be healthier, but somehow struggle with putting it all together and sustaining long-term change.

So, I imagine that you have picked up this book because you want to make lasting changes in your lifestyle. Perhaps you want to lose weight – and there is a particular focus on losing and managing weight in this book. But, as most of us know by now, while being wise about our food choices is central to health, keeping moving and living a balanced life is also vitally important, and I cover these in lots of detail too.

I am tired of reading faddy health books that will only be followed by those who are obsessed with restrictive eating plans or complicated fitness routines. Of course, there is useful information in some of these books, but I know that most people with busy lives don't have the time or inclination to follow these as long-term strategies for maintaining their weight, fitness and well-being. And it's the long term that interests me: if you can develop the right habits you can do a lot to prevent lifestyle health issues – from your teens right up to your nineties!

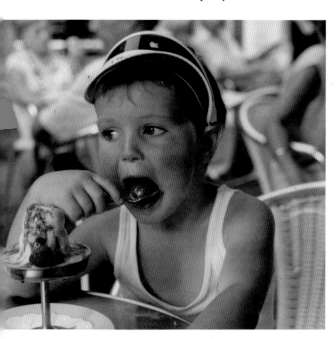

From experience, I know that my approach to diet, fitness and wellbeing is effective. When I say 'from experience' I'm not just talking about the work I've done with clients. I'm talking about my life. As many people know, I grew up in a gym environment, as my dad, Pat Henry, opened his gym in 1986 when I was four years old. I was there before school, after school and basically any time I wasn't in school. And yet I was a child and teen who was last around the pitch when playing sports. I was not naturally fit and had to work really hard on controlling my weight and staying active. And when I got to college, my eating habits were typical of a young guy living away from home for the first time – I lived on takeaways! My wake-up call will be familiar to many people: I saw a photograph of myself and was a bit horrified by the bloated face staring out at me. More about this on page 67.

I am not a naturally thin person. While I'm tall, my natural build is stocky and prone to gaining weight. So I have to work hard to stay at a healthy weight. Luckily, my job keeps me very active, but I take nothing for granted and I know that if I was sitting at a desk or driving a car all day, it would be an ongoing challenge to remain at a healthy weight and be fit (a challenge that would be doable, though, as I know from working with clients – this book is all about helping you to meet the challenge, whatever your natural make-up and circumstances).

Having just been negative about people getting obsessed with their diet and fitness programmes, I have to admit to getting obsessed myself sometimes – for instance, training for an Ironman challenge and getting so 'in the zone' that I start to irritate everyone around me. In other words, I am not perfect and I know that finding the right balance doesn't come easily to anyone. So even though I'm seen as being very fit and the expert with all the answers, I have had to get to grips with lots of issues myself over the years, and I continue to work on them.

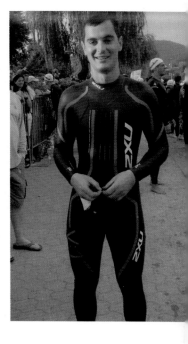

I have my good days and my bad days. I know just how hard it is to live in a balanced way, and apart from lots of information on diet, fitness and general wellbeing, I am sharing all the tips and tricks that I have discovered to make healthier living as easy as possible.

I started personal training when I was a 19-year-old student, travelling to clients' homes to do personal-training sessions. I have done over 25,000 sessions with clients since! (That's an average of 30 to 40 personal training sessions weekly over 17 years.) The work has expanded over the years into newspaper columns, books, radio and TV – with over a decade of Operation Transformation on RTÉ – and into work with businesses, developing health and fitness programmes for their staff. It has been an incredible journey, one where I am learning every day, trying new campaigns and new ways of motivating people.

The thing about all this experience is this: I have learned from every mistake that there is. I have seen diet and fitness trends come and go. Sometimes the trends bring useful new insights into how the body works or have a lasting effect. But parts of the health and fitness business have become so over the top, so obsessive and, frankly, so bound up in a fake idea of attractiveness and what it means to be healthy that it's a turn-off for those who actually need to get healthy the most.

I am far more excited about your potential for change by following the advice in this book than I would be giving you some quick-fix programme.

When I hear about some 'revolutionary' new diet, just like you, I have to cut through all the noise to figure out what's credible. Through everything I've experienced, both personally and in my work with clients, and through everything I've read about nutrition and learned from the experts I've worked with, I have concluded that when it comes to fixing a weight issue, there are no shortcuts. But that does not mean that eating healthily is not straightforward.

It saddens me to see faddy stuff taking hold, because it's making healthy eating far more complicated than it needs to be and putting people off. Not only that, it is bad for people's relationship with food when they feel that eating is a minefield and something to be feared, rather than a source of nourishment and enjoyment, as it should be.

So the purpose of this book is for it to be something you can use regardless of your current weight or fitness level. I have learned that a consistent approach is the one sure-fire way of losing weight, building fitness and becoming healthier. If that sounds a bit underwhelming, it shouldn't. I am actually far more excited about your potential for change by following the advice in this book than I would be at giving you some quick-fix programme. That's because I know that everything in this book will fit into your life. And the beauty of it is that because you are building up your knowledge and confidence – discovering that you can try new things, develop new skills and build new habits – it's an approach that will become second nature and remain with you for life.

I am 36 now and my body is totally different to how it was in my twenties. It reacts differently to various training methods than it used to, it takes longer to get a result and sometimes the result isn't what I expected! I say this to make the point that if a full-time fitness professional is always being surprised and having to tweak things, then you shouldn't be surprised either by how your body reacts to change. Part of the beauty of taking a broad-based approach to diet and fitness is getting to know your body very well and being able to work with it at every stage and age.

I've called this a handbook and I hope you can treat it like that – a friendly, easy-to-follow guide that will bring you on a journey, page by page, chapter by chapter. You'll find that some themes and advice come up a few times – that's because I want to get across some key ideas that are the bedrock of a healthy lifestyle. You will be amazed at just how easy it is to make straightforward changes and what a difference they can make. Not only that, the benefits of feeling healthier and more active will help you stay on course and motivate you to keep going. My ambition is to help you realize that losing weight and getting fitter can be simple – so simple that you can't not start, no matter how small that start is!

I hope you can treat this like a friendly, easy-to-follow guide that will bring you on a journey, page-by-page, chapter-by-chapter.

1 THE FIRST STEP

Before you start, I want you to sit down somewhere quiet and do a bit of thinking about what you're about to do and why. There are complicated answers to why people become overweight and unfit – entire books and lengthy academic papers have been written on the topic. But the simple answer – and the one that makes sense for this book – is: life! At times, life itself just gets in the way and before you know it you have started to put on weight, sit more, stop exercising and become unhealthy. It can happen to the best of us and you are certainly not alone.

On top of that, all the talk in the media about the 'obesity crisis' can make it feel like it's a plague that's out of control and you are helpless. It's certainly the case that modern living – industrialized food production, wall-to-wall advertising, faddy food advice, long commutes, high-stress living – makes it harder to make good lifestyle choices. My aim in this book is to give you the tools to make better choices, even with all those pressures, and to help you understand that actually it's not that complicated. I hope you'll gain a sense of ownership about your health. And the journey starts with having a heart-to-heart with yourself about where you are now and what you want to do about it.

The idea of this first step is to assess the now – where you are and where you want to go, to see what health means to you and what has stopped you making good choices in the past. Going through

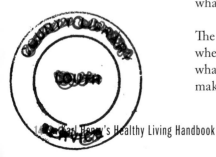

these questions will help you become firm in your resolution to make lasting changes.

The questions may seem basic, but give them a little thought. You might even think the 'yes/no' questions are a bit obvious, but be totally honest with yourself. Knowing where you are in your head will go a long way towards helping you to succeed in becoming healthier. It will show you if you are torn between wanting to do the right thing and believing there is something preventing you from doing so.

And if you feel there are obstacles to making changes in your life, I'd challenge you to think about whether they are genuine or whether your fear of failure is even greater than your desire to be healthier. Maybe you tried diets or lifestyle changes in the past that were not practical for your circumstances or were too extreme and impossible to maintain?

If you are doubtful about your ability to change, I'd encourage you to look through this book. You'll see that nothing I am suggesting is beyond you, and apart from practical information about food, fitness and living more healthily, there are lots of tips and tools to motivate and support you. Once you've had a look through and had time to think about it more deeply, I hope you will be able to complete this section.

Taking the time to look at your mindset and to identify what health means to you is one of the simplest ways of jumpstarting your thinking. This is both a contract with yourself and the foundation of a new approach to living.

...the journey starts with having a heart-to-heart with yourself about where you are now and what you want to do about it.

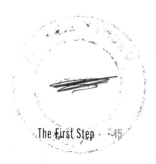

YOUR CONTRACT

WHAT DOES HEALTH MEAN TO YOU? TRY TO COME UP WITH FIVE MEANINGS:

1. _____
2. _____
3. _____
4. _____
5. _____

ARE YOU WILLING TO MAKE CHANGES TO YOUR LIFE TO START GETTING HEALTHY?

YES ☐   NO ☐

LIST THREE REASONS WHY YOU HAVEN'T BEEN ABLE TO MAKE THOSE CHANGES ALREADY:

1. _____
2. _____
3. _____

WERE THESE REASONS TRULY HOLDING YOU BACK?

YES ☐   NO ☐

ARE YOU READY TO STOP MAKING EXCUSES FOR NOT BEING ABLE TO LOSE WEIGHT AND GET HEALTHY?

YES ☐   NO ☐

ARE YOU READY TO STOP LOOKING FOR A QUICK-FIX SOLUTION?

YES ☐   NO ☐

NOW THAT YOU KNOW THAT YOU WANT TO BE HEALTHIER, WHAT ARE YOU WILLING TO CHANGE AND PRIORITIZE TO MAKE THOSE GOALS HAPPEN? LIST FIVE THINGS (OR MORE!):

1. _____

2. _____

3. _____

4. _____

5. _____

WELL DONE ON TAKING THE FIRST STEP TO ACHIEVING YOUR HEALTH GOALS! NOW, WHY DON'T YOU SIGN BELOW? MAKE A PROMISE TO YOURSELF THAT FROM THIS DAY FORWARD YOU ARE COMMITTED TO MAKING LASTING CHANGES.

SIGNATURE
_____

DATE
_____

2 GET THE MEASURE OF YOURSELF

Every January, people trying to lose weight make a New Year's resolution to follow a new diet. Very often it tends to be a quick-fix solution involving the latest trend. While there may be changes, they tend to be short-lived and inevitably the weight creeps back on. This generally happens for three reasons:

1. **Whatever the fix, it was unsustainable** and just set you up to fail from the very start. Yet you feel guilty having failed. Don't! It was never going to last.

2. **You didn't spend time assessing the now** – what caused you to get into an unhealthy rut and how it got to the stage you're at. Spending time analysing the real reasons for being overweight and/or unfit is crucial to your long-term health, as you can learn from your mistakes.

3. **You didn't measure things.** By measuring different aspects of health, you will see progress. And progress leads to change, which leads to increased motivation. It's a virtuous cycle of effort and motivation.

These are the three most common reasons that I see all the time. But I'm going to focus on the third one here, because I think it's possibly the most important tool you have when trying to achieve long-lasting change.

When you think about it, there are very few businesses that don't give their staff targets. Why? Because targets give people something to work towards, a reason for getting out of bed and going into work; they are a measure of achievement.

On a personal level, how many people actually set goals or targets? What were yours when you last tried to get healthy? Or did you decide in a vague way that you wanted to 'lose weight' or 'get healthier', or even 'drop two stone by the summer', started trying but fell off the wagon after a few weeks as you got bored or didn't really notice any difference (except maybe a few pounds off the scales – but not enough to make the level of effort seem worthwhile or to keep you motivated).

While being clear about what went wrong in the past and why you want to make changes is crucial, once you have done that, you need to set targets and measure your progress. Measuring things consistently will keep you healthy for the rest of your life. When you have a bad day, it keeps you focused, and knowing where you are against your targets reduces the chances of you falling off the wagon in the long-term too.

I know the thought of measuring your current fitness and health may be a little scary – after all, there's nowhere to hide from the black-and-white numbers, and the recommended guidelines for weight and waistlines are so low that they seem unachievable. But there is no need to be scared – I will guide you through the various key measurements and give you the real numbers that you need to know to make them a helpful tool in losing weight and getting healthier.

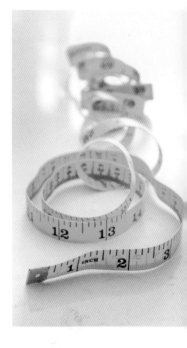

Once you measure some element of your fitness every week, you will begin to see the benefits of all your hard work. Whether it's from the improvements in your food or from doing extra exercise, once you see the numbers going in the right direction, you will become even more motivated and positive.

And don't forget: no matter what your starting numbers are, once you begin to bring them down, you are getting healthier!

What I am proposing is that on Day 1 you measure one of three things, or even all three if you want. Then every week, at the same time, on the same day, you measure again. A week is long enough to see the changes having an effect. Measuring at the same time is essential – ideally in the morning, as in the evening you will be heavier, more bloated and have a higher resting heart rate. (A classic gym trick is to measure yourself initially in the evening and then a few weeks later in the morning. The big variance in the results will make any changes that have happened look more dramatic than they really are!)

No matter what your starting numbers are, once you begin to bring them down, you are getting healthier!

Let's take a look at what you can measure. Remember, you don't have to measure everything – just measure what you feel is the most doable for you.

RESTING HEART RATE

Your resting heart rate is one of the most effective ways of measuring your fitness. Ideally this should be taken in the morning, before getting out of bed, as your body is at its most relaxed and there are no stimulants or sugar in the body that could spike your heart rate.

The reason I love this measure is that while there are lots of complicated tests out there, this one is free and simple to do. Simply find your pulse at the base of the wrist or at the side of your neck, just under your jawline. It may be faint at first but with practice, you will find it more quickly. Now just count the beats for 15 seconds and then multiply the number of beats by 4. This gives you your resting heart rate in beats per minute (BPM).

For most of the population, the lower your resting heart rate, the healthier you are. A normal resting heart rate could be anywhere from 60 to 80 BPM. There is a very small percentage of people who will naturally have a very high or very low resting heart rate, but generally this is a good rule of thumb. (If your resting heart rate is in the nineties or over 100, I recommend a visit to your GP for a check-up and also to ease into any exercise routine gradually.)

Keep a little notepad beside your bed just to jot down your weekly BPM. Write down your Day 1 BPM straightaway and then just record the number once a week.

As you get fitter, your heart becomes stronger – actually thickening on one side of the heart wall – and works more efficiently. The fitter you are, the more efficiently the heart works.

If you want a number to aim for, ideally you should be aiming for a heart rate of 50- or 60-something BPM. But the real answer is that once it's coming down, that's a sign that your food changes and exercise are making a big difference to your body, internally as well as externally. And once you see the numbers changing and improving, you will be more focused, more motivated and more determined than ever.

Remember, you don't have to measure everything - just measure what you feel is the most doable for you.

WAIST

Your waistline is probably the most important measurement you can take. It gives you lots of information and will come down quickly with some hard work. It's the simplest to measure, but also the scariest for so many people. Perhaps because there is no place to hide from it!

There are two types of fat that we store: the fat you can pinch with your fingers and then the dangerous

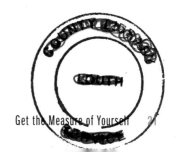

internal fat that you can't pinch – visceral fat. Visceral fat is deep inside the body, behind the abdominal wall, and it surrounds your internal organs.

Waist size is a pretty good guide to the amount of fat that is lurking in there. We can link a high waistline measurement to a huge number of medical conditions. Many women are annoyed by having big hips, but fat on the hips is mainly just under the skin, and is healthier than fat around the midriff, which may be interfering with the organs. On the other hand, having a lot of visceral fat is actually dangerous and that's why waist size is so important.

The best way to measure your body fat is by having a DEXA scan, but that's time-consuming and expensive. Alternatively, you can weigh yourself on body composition scales, but unless you have medical-standard Tanita scales like we have in our gym, you won't be getting an accurate reading. Or you can get a trained professional to use body calipers to measure your fat levels. The simple two-euro solution is to use a tape measure – you'll get the key information you need without the hassle or cost of the more complex methods.

The simple two-euro solution to measuring your body fat is to use a tape measure!

People get confused about where their waist actually is. Your waist is not your jean or trouser size or the narrowest part of your torso if you're a woman with curves. Instead, use your belly button as your guide for where to measure – it is a visual indicator that will be in the same spot for the rest of your life! Simply take the tape measure and put it around your mid-section at the same level all round, meeting at your belly button. This is your waist.

The Safefood guidelines for a healthy waist measurement are not greater than 80cm/32in for women and not greater than 94cm/37in for men. I feel these are a little low and even counterproductive, as they can seem unattainable and can turn people off measuring their waist at all.

Just remember, no matter what number you get, by getting it down, you are getting healthier. Certainly you should be looking to get your number down into the thirties, as when your waistline is above 40 inches you are in the high-risk category for so many medical conditions, such as cardiovascular disease, metabolic disorders and diabetes. But the reality is that the closer you can get it to the recommended guidelines, the healthier you are and once you begin to measure it, that is a start in itself. And if you make simple changes to your diet and introduce exercise into your day, you will see a consistent fall in your waist measurement.

Again, try to measure your waist once a week at the same time on the same day.

WEIGHT

This is the measurement you probably expected me to start with! But I think the first two are more important. Still, there is no denying that pounds and stones or kilos* is what everyone thinks of when it comes to health, and for people who really get into it, they look further to see what their body is composed of – how much is fat tissue and how much is lean tissue (e.g. muscle).

I believe that it's worthwhile to measure your weight consistently. With constant measurement, you will notice if you're gaining weight before it becomes an issue and can rectify it with healthy eating and exercise. Weigh in once a week, ideally first thing in the morning, and keep a note of your weight so you can measure your progress. If you are following this

It is worthwhile to measure your weight consistently – you will notice if you're gaining weight before it becomes an issue.

---

* 1lb = 0.45kg; 1kg = 2.2lbs; 1 stone (14lbs) = 6.3kg

book, you will see it go down (and as you won't be building a lot of muscle by following any of my plans, you won't be replacing the weight of the lost fat by a huge amount of muscle tissue).

Hopping on the scales is sufficient for most people – you're keeping an eye on the overall direction of your weight. However, you aren't getting a measure of the make-up of your weight, whether it's fat or muscle. For most people, this isn't important – you simply want to see your weight going down as you eat a healthier diet and exercise more. And if you are eating better and becoming fitter, you will be losing excess body fat and improving your ratio of lean to fat tissue.

For health, you don't need to be training hard and making big lean tissue gains.

For health, you don't need to be training hard and making big lean tissue gains. For appearance, though, many people get into heavy training. Remember that 1lb of tissue – either fat or muscle – is 1lb. The weight is identical. But because muscle tissue is denser, it takes up less space than fat, so people who have more muscle than fat have a more streamlined appearance. Any weight-bearing exercise (e.g. walking) will improve the amount of lean tissue you have on your body.

There is one further thing to consider – unfortunately, for a variety of biological reasons, we naturally store more fat as we get older. In other words, someone who is eating exactly the same diet and has the same level of activity in their fifties as in their twenties is going to lay down more fat simply because of the hormonal changes that come with age. The good news is that exercise plays a key role in slowing down and even reversing this process, helping to keep more lean tissue on your body.

To get you started, you might want to use this table to keep track of your key measurements:

	RESTING HEART RATE	WAIST	WEIGHT
WEEK 1 DATE: __/__/____			
WEEK 2 DATE: __/__/____			
WEEK 3 DATE: __/__/____			
WEEK 4 DATE: __/__/____			
WEEK 5 DATE: __/__/____			
WEEK 6 DATE: __/__/____			
WEEK 7 DATE: __/__/____			
WEEK 8 DATE: __/__/____			

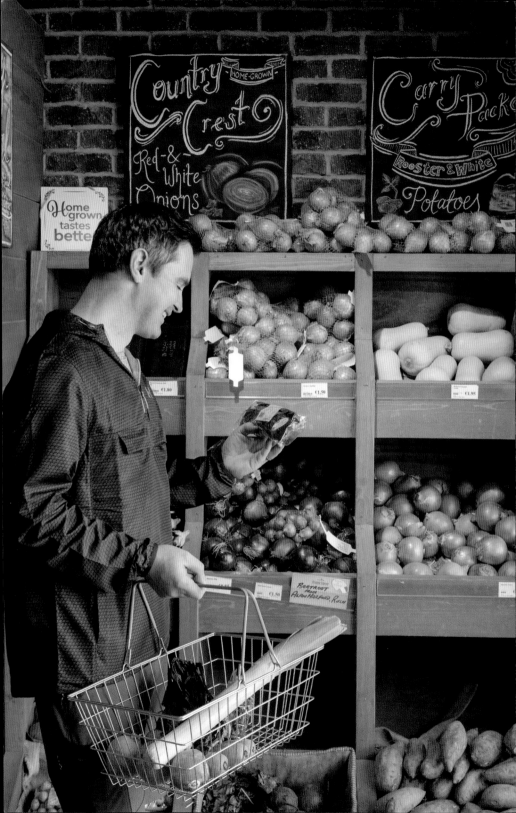

Food

What we eat and put into our bodies has the biggest impact on our health, more than anything else we do.

3 WHAT IS FOOD?

It may seem like an odd question, but maybe if we thought a bit more about what food actually is, it would help us to make better choices. What we eat and put into our bodies has the biggest impact on our health, more than anything else we do.
Over the past 70 years, how we make food has changed dramatically. Indeed, what we call food has changed an incredible amount. These changes have had a huge effect on our bodies. So it's time to go back to basics.

Food may be many things to you – a way of looking after yourself and your family or friends, a source of enjoyment, a passion even. Or it may be a chore and a source of anxiety and stress. But, of course, before any of these things, food is a biological necessity: we have to eat. And here is what food delivers to our bodies …

CALORIES

At the most basic level, food is fuel for the body. The unit of measurement for that fuel is the calorie. A calorie represents the amount of energy (or fuel) released to the body when food is consumed.

Different foods have different concentrations of energy. Gram for gram, there are far fewer calories in, say, an apple than a chocolate bar, so your body gets less fuel from an apple than a chocolate bar of the same weight. The main reason for putting on excess weight is taking in more fuel than the body can make use of – then, depending on the source of the calorie, it just puts the unused fuel into storage as fat.

The government recommendations for daily calorie intake are 2,500 calories for a man and 2,000 calories for a woman. The ideal calorie intake can vary, though, depending on your age, your size, your inbuilt metabolic rate (some people have naturally slower engines than others and there is only a limited amount you can do to change that) and your activity levels during the day (there is a lot you can do about that, as I explain in this book).

The number of calories you need will also depend on your body composition. Remember, we talked about body composition in the last section – the ratio of lean tissue (muscle) to fat tissue that makes up your body. It's better to have a higher ratio of lean tissue because it burns more calories than fat tissue. Again, you can do a lot to shift that ratio as you lose weight (reduce fat tissue) and get more active (increase lean tissue).

A further consideration when it comes to health is that not all calories are equal – while 100 calories from fresh vegetables and 100 calories from a couple of biscuits are identical amounts of fuel for the body, the vegetables have lots more going on in terms of nutrients, such as vitamins and minerals and fibre, that do great things for your system. They are nutrition multitaskers, not just providing fuel but also keeping the engine running smoothly. On the other hand, the biscuits will only pump out energy and do nothing to help your body stay lively, tuned up and running well.

When it comes to health, not all calories are equal ... nutritionally, vegetables have lots more to offer than biscuits!

Remember, every pound of fat you lose off your body is actually 3,500 calories of energy. This is so important to remember, as 1lb is actually a huge number of calories; if you can lose that each week, it's 4lbs per month or 52lbs in a year.

	15 MINUTES	30 MINUTES	1 HOUR
WALKING	91	182	364
CYCLING	160	320	640
RUNNING	180	360	720
SWIMMING	120	240	480
RESISTANCE TRAINING	91	182	364
HOUSEWORK	72	144	288

To get you thinking about the relationship between calories and energy expenditure, the table above shows the average numbers of calories used up in doing different exercises across three time periods. These numbers will obviously vary with factors such as age, fitness, metabolic rate, weight, body composition and overall health, but this table will give you a simple picture of how the body uses calories.

PROTEIN

Protein is a substance that helps to build and repair the body. It helps to repair your muscles after exercise and can be great for your immune system too.

Protein is contained mainly in meat, fish, eggs and other dairy produce, nuts and seeds, and occurs in lower levels in all kinds of beans and pulses.

Protein is incredibly important for your body, and generally we don't eat enough of it. Normally I get my clients to make two of their three daily meals protein-based. You should aim to eat 1.5g of protein per kilo (2.2lbs) of your weight. When it comes to meat, ideally focus on lean white proteins.

CARBOHYDRATES

We've said already that calories are a measure of energy. Now we come to carbohydrates, which are an important source of energy. (Of course, all foods are a source of energy, but this is the distinctive characteristic of carbohydrates.) Carbohydrates supply energy for your muscles and fuel your day.

Carbohydrate foods are staples like bread, pasta, rice, potatoes and beans and pulses (again – beans and pulses have good levels of both protein and carbohydrates). You also get carbs in smaller quantities in most vegetables, but particularly root vegetables like carrots, parsnips and sweet potatoes.

You are better off choosing wholegrain versions of breads, pastas and grains because the white versions are very refined, which means most of the nutrients and fibre have been stripped away. You should normally be taking in 200g to 300g of good-quality carbohydrates per day.

SUGARS

On food labels, sugar is usually listed as a subsection of, or beneath, carbohydrates, because sugar is a form of carbohydrate (the ones I mentioned earlier are starches). Sugar is like rocket fuel for your body – something that provides it with a big surge of energy. But if you're not going to use that energy for a lot of activity, it's only going to go into storage. I have more to say about how to keep an eye on how much sugar you're eating further along in this chapter and will be talking about sugar in more detail in the next chapter.

FATS

The fat you carry if you are overweight isn't simply excess fat (butter, oil, lard, etc.) that you ate over

Choose wholegrain versions of breads, pastas and grains because the white versions are very refined which means most of the nutrients have been stripped away.

the years and nothing else. How your body deals with excess fuel and lays down fat stores is more complicated than that! So you don't need to be more afraid of fat than any other nutrient. Indeed, fats are crucial for us to have healthy bodies. We need fats in moderation to function properly and they help us absorb other nutrients. However, not all fats are created equal. There are good fats, bad fats and fats the experts are still debating:

Monounsaturated fats

From sources like oils (e.g. olive, rapeseed), nuts and avocados. These are good fats.

Polyunsaturated fats

From oils, nuts and seeds, similar to monounsaturated fats. Polyunsaturated fats include omega-3 fats that are found in high quantities in oily fish such as salmon and mackerel. These are also good fats.

Saturated fats

Most associated with meat and dairy products such as butter, but also high in things like chocolate and coconut oil. These used to be considered bad for us, but now many reputable scientists say they're not so bad. Like lots of debates in the field of nutrition, it turns out that there is no 'one size fits all' approach – our bodies are too complex for that.

Trans fats

These are industrial fats that are used mainly in the manufacture of processed foods but are also sold as margarine and butter-substitute spreads. They do not occur in nature, which tells you all you need to know about them. They are bad fats that you should avoid.

FOOD LABELS

Knowledge is power, and when it comes to eating healthily, understanding food labels is a useful skill.

You are more likely to make the best choices if you can interpret the information on food packaging. Once you've got the basics, you can pick up any product anywhere and know if it's a good option or if it's wiser to put it back on the shelf.

If I was to give you a shortcut for making decisions when reading food labels, it would be to search for a product's sugar content and see how many grams of sugar it contains per serving. Ideally this number should be as low as possible.

Begin to look at the foods you are eating and aim for ones that have a low amount of sugar. You will be amazed at just how much sugar is in the foods that you eat. There are 4g of sugar in a teaspoon, so you can easily work out how many teaspoons of sugar there are in a serving of a product – just divide the number of grams of sugar per serving by four to tell you the number of teaspoons. You probably wouldn't sprinkle spoonful after spoonful of sugar over a bowl of pasta or a plate of curry, and yet you might discover that a tomato or curry sauce you are buying contains eight or nine teaspoons of sugar per serving.

Apart from trans fats, you don't have to get into a sweat about which fats to avoid. Eating a range of real foods, and not eating too much of anything, will have you on the right track. To avoid trans fats, knowing what to look for on a label is essential. Look out for the word 'hydrogenated' – hydrogenated or partially hydrogenated oils are trans fats. If you see that word on a jar or packet, put it back on the shelf.

Another thing you should watch out for on labels is salt content. Too much salt is bad for us – particularly for our blood pressure – and a lot of the salt we eat comes from processed food (including staples like bread and breakfast cereals). Salt on labels is usually listed as sodium. If the measure is given in grams, multiply that number by 2.5 to get the equivalent amount of salt.

If I was to give you a shortcut for making decisions when reading food labels, it would be to search for a product's sugar content ...

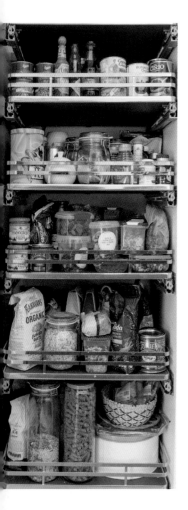

If it's in milligrams, you'll have to divide by 1,000 first and then multiply by 2.5. The usual guideline health authorities give is that we shouldn't eat more than 6g of salt per day (and that includes salt you add yourself in cooking or serving your dinner). As 6g of salt is about 1 teaspoon, you can see how easy it is to overdo it.

Labels may also include a lot of information about other nutrients (perhaps in the hope that you won't notice all the additives they contain). Again, if you're eating a broad range of foods, you can be assured that you're getting a variety of nutrients and you don't need to sweat the small stuff.

If there is a long list of additives on a label – particularly additives that sound like they belong in a science lab – that's a signal that the food is very processed and not as nutritious as it might be. Putting a lot of foods like these into your body is a bit like putting dodgy diesel into a car – while they will keep you going, you are more likely to keep the engine running smoothly over time if you simply don't do it too often.

Of course, if you can develop your cookery skills, the number of labels you will need to read will diminish, because it's mainly processed foods that have complicated labels. You don't usually see long-winded information in tiny type on the side of a banana, a bag of nuts or a piece of chicken!

There's a recipe section further on that will give you some simple meal ideas to get you going. Cooking really isn't that complicated and you don't need to have gone to a cookery school or be at MasterChef level to be able to feed yourself and your family healthy, tasty and budget-friendly food. And if you're worried about time, there are lots of quick recipes and things you can cook in bulk and then freeze so that you have your own homemade ready-meals, available in a matter of minutes when you come in from work.

Top tips for identifying good foods

- ☐ Foods that don't need labels.

- ☐ Foods that you need to cook yourself.

- ☐ Foods with a short shelf life.

- ☐ Foods that don't have added sugars.

- ☐ Foods that are high in fibre.

- ☐ Foods that are high in good fats.

- ☐ Foods that are low in added salt.

- ☐ Foods without words like 'diet', 'low fat' or 'fat-free' on the label.

- ☐ Lean forms of protein.

- ☐ Plain water with no added flavours.

- ☐ All vegetables and particularly green vegetables.

- ☐ Unprocessed nuts and seeds.

- ☐ Local meat, fish, grains, fruit and veg.

4 MAKE FRIENDS WITH CARBS

In the last chapter, I said food is energy and calories are a measure of energy. Well, a more sophisticated way of measuring food's effect on our body is to look at what happens when it is broken down by digestion, ready to be used as fuel. The fuel takes the form of blood sugars (glucose) in the blood stream. So nutritionists measure the impact of various foods according to their glycaemic index (GI)* – in other words, how fast they cause the level of blood sugars to rise.

I also said in the last chapter that the particular role of carbohydrates is to supply us with energy. So the glycaemic index applies mainly to carbohydrates. Different carbohydrates will cause blood sugars to increase (spike) at different rates – from very quickly to very slowly and everything in between. The ideal is to have a steady level of blood sugars for a few hours after eating, rather than a big spike and then a crash.

When your blood sugars are steady, you will feel alert, positive, happy and be able to work hard. Consistent levels of blood sugars result in consistent levels of energy, mood and concentration.

When your blood sugars rise quickly and then crash, you will struggle to concentrate, feel unproductive and sluggish and find your mood dipping.

---

* Glycaemia literally means 'sugar in the blood', from the words 'glyco' (sugar) and 'aemia' (a word for anything to do with the blood.

Following on from this, you can see that low GI foods are better for you than high GI foods. High GI foods more often than not…

- are high in sugar and additives
- are highly processed
- are processed foods that you don't have to prepare
- have 'fat-free', 'low fat', 'diet' or 'no added sugar' on the label
- have a long shelf life

On the other hand, low GI foods…

- are less processed or refined – brown foods such as brown bread, brown pasta, brown rice
- have a short shelf life
- are foods that you have to prepare or cook yourself
- are in season

THE VICIOUS SUGAR CIRCLE

The highest GI food is sugar. While there are natural sugars in things like fruit, root vegetables (like carrots and beetroot) and milk, the kinds I'm talking about are those that are processed and added to all kinds of foods, including savoury.

As I said in the previous chapter, sugar is like rocket fuel for the body – it's a pure form of energy that gives you a big rush when it hits your bloodstream. It's bad for your stomach, your teeth and your weight (our bodies store it as fat once we have used what we need as fuel), yet it is so hard to get rid of as it's addictive and the sugar rush can make you feel good.

What is happening when you feel a craving for a Danish pastry or a chocolate biscuit in the morning or in the afternoon is that your blood sugar levels are dropping. They drop quickly after the initial rush from high-sugar foods (such as a breakfast or lunch

…sugar is like rocket fuel for the body - it's a pure form of energy that gives you a big rush when it hits your bloodstream.

comprised of processed foods) and the sugar crash makes you crave more high-sugar foods. It's a vicious circle: the more sugar you consume, the more you need in order to feel OK and keep going. Your body has become addicted to sugar and wants more of it all the time.

Remember what I said about reading labels, and how surprised you would be to realize just how much sugar is in the foods that we eat? It is in most processed foods, often under a less familiar name – any ingredient with '-ose' at the end of it (e.g. glucose, dextrose) is a sugar. Fructose and lactose are natural sugars (and fine in their natural form in fruit and milk), while some of the others are man-made.

Sweeteners may not have the calories of sugar, but scientists have found their effects on the body to be similar to the real thing.

Just as bad as sugar are manufactured sweeteners such as aspartame, which is even more processed than sugar itself. Sweeteners may not have the calories of sugar, but scientists have found their chemical effects on the body to be very similar to the real thing. Put simply, they don't stop you being addicted to the sweet stuff!

Changing your diet to reduce your sugar intake is hard. But while it is a tough habit to break, once you stick with it for a few days, you will feel and be healthier and happier.

WHITE FOODS

Moving on from sugar, I always summarize high GI foods as 'white foods' – things like white bread, white pasta, white rice and mashed potatoes. These high GI foods are all carbohydrates that have been refined – meaning that they've been heavily processed or radically changed from their natural state. For instance, husks and skins have been removed and with them the fibre that slows down digestion. Or the starch molecules in the potatoes have been broken up in the action of mashing. They are now made up of small, soft particles that are broken down in the body really quickly and are ready to hit your bloodstream.

Low GI carbs are less refined. It takes the body more effort to break them down and for their energy to be released. Therefore their effect on the blood isn't instant. These carbohydrates won't cause your blood sugars to shoot up quickly and then drop just as rapidly. Instead, they'll deliver a steady stream of energy. By eating these foods at regular intervals, you will have more focus and a better mood. And you will be fuller for longer and less tempted to snack on processed foods.

Unfortunately, the typical Irish diet is full of high GI carbohydrates. But the answer is not to cut out carbs. I am not anti-carbohydrates like so many people writing about food and nutrition – I am mad about carbs, the healthy low GI ones!

Sources of low GI carbohydrates include porridge, low GI granola and all the brown foods. Indeed, switching from white to brown is the easiest thing you can do to make a big difference to your wellbeing in a short space of time. Make that toast, sandwich, pasta or rice wholegrain or brown. When it comes to breads, aim for those that are harder and full of nuts and seeds too. Wholegrain and wholemeal carbs are full of fibre and other nutrients, aiding your digestive system and internal organs too. (You can find plenty more about what foods are low GI by simply looking up 'low GI foods' online.)

Carbohydrates are not the enemy; it's just the processed ones.

Carbohydrates are not the enemy; it's just the processed ones. Aim to get the best version that you can – and they don't have to be expensive. For example, in Ireland, we have some fantastic oatmeal producers whose produce is in its natural state, competitively priced, local and extremely good for you.

5 BE GUT AWARE

In the last few years, you may have noticed far more articles and books about 'gut health' – which is a polite way of talking about the journey food makes from your dinner plate to your toilet bowl, and what happens inside your body on that journey!

The health of your gut is crucial to how you look, feel and get through the day, yet traditionally most of us have paid little attention to it. We looked elsewhere – to tablets and supplements, to products that masked problems rather than solved them. It is great that gut health is now a hot topic, because the digestive process is a really important part of total health.

Your gut is directly linked to your brain, and between the two, they control everything that you do and want. And if you get stressed or worried, your digestive system is one of the first parts of the body to be affected. Digestion is all about how your body absorbs the nutrients from food. And there is a lot you can do to improve digestive health:

SLOW DOWN YOUR EATING AND CHEW

We eat so fast now that our stomachs have a hard time processing the food, putting a huge strain on the whole digestive system. The simplest way to remedy this is to put down your knife and fork for about 15 to 20 seconds between each bite of food and chew thoroughly. This improves digestion as the food is more broken down before it enters your stomach and the stomach has less to do. It will also give the nerves in your stomach lining time to register the presence of food and tell your brain when you're full. It takes about 20 minutes for the message to get through. If you eat too quickly, you may be still eating when you're already full; your brain just hasn't got the message yet!

EXERCISE MORE

Exercise, in any form, will help the body, stomach and mind. The hormones released during exercise will help your digestive system. I will be explaining more about how to create your own exercise programme later in the book, so when you get going with this, you'll know you are helping your gut as well as everything else.

REDUCE YOUR STRESS LEVELS

Stress is one of the biggest causes of stomach problems, so take a look at what stresses you out and aim to reduce it in any way you can. Easier said than done, I realize, but start with the practical stuff and figure out the complex stuff as you go along.

Is your desk/car/home full of clutter and a total mess? Chances are that this is a reflection of your own mind and is probably stressing you out, even if you don't realize it (ever wondered why you feel so good after a spring clean?). Getting places you spend time in a bit more organized will improve your stress levels.

Do you have friends who stress you out? You might need to be a bit more selfish. You can still be supportive, but don't get sucked into taking on problems that you can't deal with. Avoid people who make you feel bad about yourself and try to hang out more with friends who are positive and give you a lift.

Stress is one of the biggest causes of stomach problems, so take a look at what stresses you out and aim to reduce it in any way you can.

If you have big things going on in your life that are an ongoing worry – job loss, illness in your family, financial problems – you'll find that eating better and exercising will increase resilience and help you manage your stress levels. And that will improve your gut health, which will in turn help your energy levels and ability to keep up the good work. It's all a virtuous circle!

GUT BACTERIA

Putting it simply, you have good and bad bacteria in your gut and you want to increase the good and reduce the bad. Good bacteria feed on a healthy, varied, wholefood diet. Bad bacteria feed on sugar, so the more sugar in your diet, the greater the number of bad bacteria in your gut. You want to increase the healthy, good bacteria in your gut as much as possible, as they are now understood to affect a huge range of health issues – everything from the obvious (digesting your food properly) to the less obvious (your immune system and your mood). Here are some simple ways that you can do it:

Drink a mug of warm water with a few slices of lemon in the morning before breakfast. This is one of the oldest tips ever, but it's fantastic for the body, for the skin and for your digestion.

Aim to include more brown carbohydrates in your diet. The fibre will act as a cleanser for your gut as well as giving you more energy.

Eat natural and Greek yoghurt. It is full of gut-friendly bacteria and some good fats too. But steer clear of the flavoured ones – they have a lot of added sugar. If you want to flavour your yoghurt, add some chopped fruit.

Increase your vegetable intake. Vegetables are great for the gut, especially the green ones. Some people may find certain vegetables, such as onions, don't agree with them, causing bloating and gas. You will find this out by trial and error. (Eating fermented foods can help with bloating and gas if this is a problem for you. Yoghurt fits the bill, but there are also things like sauerkraut, kimchi and kefir – traditional foods that are trendy now because of the focus on gut health and are becoming widely available. They are easy and cheap to make at home too – search online for advice.)

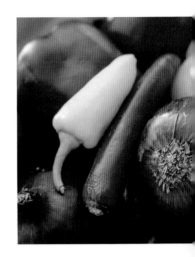

Take a good-quality digestive enzyme supplement. I don't generally recommend supplements, but if you struggle with gut health, these can be a great addition to your diet – something like Udo's Choice Super 8 Hi-Count Microbiotics or Udo's Choice Digestive Enzymes. Taking these with food can drastically increase the quantity of good bacteria in your gut.

6 BREAKING BAD HABITS

Apart from affecting our weight, the food we put into our bodies has a direct impact on how we feel, work, interact and go about our day, yet it's an association that many people don't make. The good news is that what you eat is the simplest aspect of your health that you can change. And the changes can be so straightforward that you will wonder why you didn't make them sooner, particularly when you see what a difference they make to your body, mind and health.

But before talking about how to change your diet, in this chapter, I want to talk about the habits that lead people to make the wrong food choices. If you are aware of these traps and have strategies to avoid them, then making the right choices will be easier.

SHOPPING AT THE WRONG TIME

The worst time to shop is when you are hungry. Your energy levels will be low and you will crave foods that are starchy, sugary, salty and high in trans fats. These are highly processed to taste good and make you feel instantly better. This instant gratification is what causes you to want them and keep wanting them. (Indeed, these foods are so carefully engineered to give you an instant hit that food companies refer to them as having a 'bliss point'!)

When you shop hungry, you fill your basket or trolley with high-sugar convenience foods and foods you didn't plan on getting, and you will have fewer vegetables, fruit and unprocessed foods. So, probably the simplest change you can make if you want to improve the food that comes into your household is not to shop on an empty stomach.

If you don't believe me about the power the foods in your food shop have over your health, then why not sneak a peek into other people's trollies in the supermarket? I don't encourage you to be judgmental, but you'll probably notice that healthier-looking people tend to have trollies and baskets with a bigger proportion of healthier-looking foods. (Of course, the cost of food may be an issue for you, and it's true that processed foods are often cheap and seem like good value. In the longer term, of course, their effects on your health mean they are not such a great deal after all. If you do a bit of planning and shop carefully, you can include a bigger proportion of unprocessed foods.)

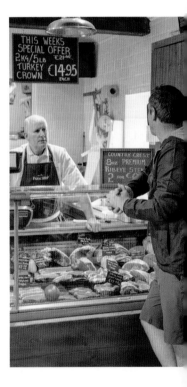

Plan to do a big food shop once a week. Planning is key. By having lots of healthy options available in the fridge, the cupboard and anywhere that you spend time during the week (your car, van or tractor, your desk, your locker, and so on), you will find it so much easier to make good choices. If you haven't planned and stocked up, then you will be chasing your tail all week and be more likely to eat takeaways and find yourself in convenience stores, getting tempted by all the packaged processed stuff. Give yourself a few hours to stock up once a week and watch the difference it makes to your life.

Here are some simple tips to help you fill the trolley as healthily as possible:

- Try to have something to eat before you go shopping – a bowl of soup, scrambled eggs or even some nuts will take the edge off your appetite and the sugary processed stuff will seem far less alluring.

- Choose foods that have a shorter shelf life – plan to eat things that only last a few days earlier in the week after your big shop and avoid anything with a very long shelf life.
- Choose foods that you have to prepare yourself.
- Choose foods with the least amount of ingredients on the label.
- Pick up lots of colourful fruit and vegetables.
- Buy fruit and veg to juice rather than prepared long-life fruit juices, which are high in sugar. Of course, water is the best drink and tap water is perfectly good. (The next chapter is all about fluids and I go into this in lots more detail.)

EMOTIONAL EATING

We have all been there: when stressed or upset, our food choices become poor and we crave high-sugar foods that make us feel better for a little while. To limit the damage from a comfort-eating binge, try these simple tips:

- Don't have foods you know you'll binge on in the house in the first place.
- Try not to shop when you're on bad form if you can possibly help it. Everything I said about shopping when hungry also applies to shopping when you're upset.
- If you're buying yourself a comfort-eating treat, get just one of the product – so just one bar instead of a whole pack.
- Plan your comfort eating i.e. decide to have a treat but limit it to just one day or one meal.
- Go for a short walk.
- Discuss your problems with a friend or partner.
- Remind yourself that it may be easy to eat but will take time to work off – (as the old saying goes, 'Seconds on the lips; a lifetime on the hips') – and you'll be annoyed with yourself later.

They may seem like really simple tips, but they work. Life is not perfect; there are good and bad days, ups and downs. It's important to accept that sometimes you're going to be in bad form and you will be near something tempting and you won't be able to resist it. That doesn't mean you're always going to do it or that you have no self-control. Don't beat yourself up about it. Remind yourself that you're taking much better care of yourself now and you are just going to resume your good habits. Draw a line in the sand and move on as quickly as you can.

MINDLESS EATING

The third pattern of behaviour that can affect your health and your waistline is mindless eating. This is where you are eating without actually thinking about it. Your focus is on something else and you are just putting food into your mouth because it is in front of you. You don't taste it, don't really chew it, and before you know it, it seems like the food has simply disappeared.

We have all been there: when stressed or upset, our food choices become poor and we crave high-sugar foods that make us feel better for a little while.

Eating while driving is a classic example of mindless eating: as your focus is on your driving (or it should be), you can eat a bag of crisps or nuts with no real recollection of doing it. Eating at your desk at work – that's another thing we are all guilty of. How often do you eat your lunch when all your attention is on your computer screen? Even if you're busy, if you can possibly break off to eat (and even better, eat and take a short walk), it will be far better for you.

Another example of mindless eating is eating in front of the TV. It's very easy for a takeaway or packet of biscuits to simply vanish, almost without you noticing, as you watch Game of Thrones.

Mindless eating has a direct link to the quantity that you eat. Eat at a table, away from your phone, your

TV and your computer and focus on the food that's on your plate, letting your mind relax as you eat.

If you have a family, eating at the table is one of the best ways to improve the family's health – new US research has found that there is a direct relationship between the quantity of time spent eating together and obesity rates within the family. Getting the family together, chatting at the table and focusing on each other is a really simple switch, but one that will have a big impact – you will be amazed at how much less you eat and how much more you enjoy your food too. (And to give your children a skill that will remain with them for life, you can have them help with preparing food and eventually cooking simple family meals themselves from time to time.)

Apart from overeating, the main issue with eating mindlessly is that you don't chew your food properly. I talked about the importance of chewing in the section on gut health. Chewing improves your digestion and the absorption of nutrients. If you focus on your food when eating, then not only will you be tasting and enjoying your food, you will also be helping your body to get more from each meal. So here are some tips to help you:

- Ask yourself if you really need or want the product.
- Don't eat when you drive or are in front of a screen.
- Eat at a table.
- Put down your knife and fork between each mouthful.
- Aim to chew your food for at least 20 seconds.
- Try to savour your food when you're eating it – think about the texture and flavour.

If you have a family, eating at the table is one of the best ways to improve the family's health ...

SUPERSIZING

The size of food portions used to be a source of fascination for visitors to the United States. Now it's a global problem and our portion sizes are far bigger than we need. Combine large portions with mindless eating and we can plough through a massive amount of food and barely even notice.

There are many studies that show that we are highly suggestible when it comes to portion sizes. We will eat what is placed in front of us – whether a big plate full of food or a medium-sized plate full of food – and consider ourselves satisfied. One study had participants reporting the same level of fullness over the course of three meals, even though the meals were getting progressively larger by 300 calories a time. (In other words, a meal that was 600 calories lower was just as satisfying as the bigger one – doesn't that make you think?)

Next time you go to the cinema, watch what food and drink people order. As often as not, they will be asked if they want to go for a larger serving. It's the same thing in fast-food restaurants. And they'll eat the lot, even though it wasn't what they set out to eat. Of course, the secret to eating at the cinema is not to eat there. Eating at the cinema is just a habit that's been fostered by cinema owners who make huge profits from selling fast food and drinks. Think of all the other activities you engage in without grazing your way through (admittedly these are becoming fewer). Just bring a bottle of water and concentrate on the film – you won't faint with hunger and you won't annoy your neighbours!

Given that we are so suggestible, we can use that to our advantage to make a healthier choice. Simply reduce the size of your plates! If you reduce your plate size by 10 per cent, you will be reducing the quantity of food that you eat. This is an especially good tool

We are highly suggestible when it comes to portion sizes - we will eat what is placed in front of us ...

if you are concerned about the quantity of food your family eats. Just change the plates, and as long as the change isn't too big, no one will notice. Ten per cent less per day is a lot less food over time.

If you really want to retrain your awareness about portion sizes and the ideal proportions of the various food groups, you can get a 'portion plate'. It's marked into segments and you fill up the plate with the indicated amount of each food. You can buy one in your local chemist or online.

DEPRIVING YOURSELF

Life is for living and you're not going to resist something you love for the rest of your life.

Don't cut out chocolate or alcohol or that pizza you love so much. When you tell yourself you can't have something, this tends to become the one thing you want. Life is for living and you're not going to resist something you love for the rest of your life. (In any case, most of these examples are only unhealthy if you eat them to excess.)

Aim for balance by having one treat meal a week and enjoying it. This is one of the most important aspects of the plans we build for our clients, and like those plans, this book is all about balance and long-term health. Allowing yourself to have a favourite meal or a few drinks creates a more balanced approach, and it will stop you from bingeing and yo-yo dieting.

So, have your treat meal and don't feel guilty about it. Schedule it in, work hard during the week, go for the very best and most natural version of it that you can and enjoy it!

YOUR DAILY DRINK

7

I simply cannot write a book on living healthily without discussing fluid and just how essential it is to kick-start the body for health and losing weight. It is one of the key areas of health that so many people forget about and neglect in their day. What you drink on a daily basis has an enormous impact on:

- your health
- your skin
- your appetite
- your energy
- your ability to concentrate
- your mental health
- your ability to train
- your recovery after training

You know how much I like to measure things! Well, you can use the simple chart on the next page to track your fluid intake for a week. Just put a little tick in the relevant box every time you drink anything. You will be amazed how much you drink of some things and how little of others.

If you have a lot of ticks in any box other than water, you need to consider rebalancing your fluid intake. Let's look at the various drinks in more detail:

Tea/coffee: These are staples and we have become incredibly reliant on them. Both contain caffeine, which is a stimulant, and will give you a kick-start to your day. One coffee a day won't do you any harm

	TEA	COFFEE	JUICES	FIZZY DRINKS	DIET DRINKS	WATER	ALCOHOL
MON							
TUES							
WED							
THURS							
FRI							
SAT							
SUN							

at all, maybe even two. With tea you could have up to three cups. But more than that I believe is too much for you. You are far better off replacing the excess with herbal teas such as peppermint or ginger. Whatever you're drinking – coffee, tea, herbal tea – go for the best quality you can. Coffee is best served black with some skimmed milk or espresso style.

Another issue is that tea and coffee breaks often include something sugary on the side, whether it's a biscuit or a chocolate bar. All these little extras add up. So aim to have your cuppa on its own and just enjoy it.

Juices: These are healthy if freshly made. The problem is that most of the juice we pick up in cartons in the supermarket has a long shelf life, so it's therefore highly pasteurized and is really just another variant of sugar that your body doesn't need. (Indeed, numerous recent reports have shown that there is as much, and sometimes more, sugar in a glass of pasteurized fruit juice than in a similar amount of a fizzy drink.)

The best way to have juice is to make it with just one piece of fruit and a few vegetables. This is a really simple tip to reduce the quantity of sugar in your juices.

Fizzy drinks: There are roughly 10 teaspoons of sugar in a normal can of carbonated drink, and roughly 15 in a 500ml bottle. This is white refined sugar that will go straight into your body for energy and eventually be stored as fat if you don't use it. As part of a balanced diet, one can of fizzy drink a week isn't a big deal. But if you are having one or two a day, that is a lot of refined sugar going into your body. Remember everything I said about sugar and how addictive it is? So if you have a fizzy-drink habit, you may find it hard to break. But it's worth it. If you take the seven-day kick-start challenge in the next chapter, that will get you going.

Diet drinks: If you want to get healthier, you should avoid anything with 'diet' on the label. Diet drinks replace sugar with aspartame, which is sweeter, cheaper and reacts similarly to sugar in your body. (Diet foods in general will have more artificial ingredients and preservatives than the product they replace, so you are better off going for the original version of the product. Take a look at the quantities of the ingredients on the label of a diet product versus the original version; there will be a lot more in the diet version. Avoid!)

Water: When I talk about the importance of fluid, I mean water, nothing else. Water is essential for health. Indeed, it is one of the superfoods – there's nothing unhealthy about it. We need it to hydrate our bodies and flush out toxins. You should be drinking between 2 and 3 litres per day. Yes, you will be going to the toilet more, but that's a good thing, as it's a sign that you are keeping yourself hydrated and looking after your liver and kidneys (they do the body's detoxing work – if you keep them happy with lots of water, you won't need to go on any complicated or expensive detox plans). That will settle in time.

Unless you live in a place where the tap water is contaminated, the water coming out of your kitchen tap is perfectly good. If you're buying water, I believe still water is better than sparkling, as the bubbles can affect some people's digestion, but any water is better than none – unless you buy one of the flavoured (i.e. sugary) varieties, which changes everything! If you want to flavour your water then add any of the following to a jug and drink through the morning or afternoon:

- a small handful of mint
- sliced-up citrus fruit – lemons, oranges or limes
- a handful of berries
- apple cider vinegar
- sliced cucumber
- melon slices
- any fruit that is close to going off
- a few thin slices of ginger

Why not dig out your fluid chart again and try to track your fluid intake, this time focusing on increasing your water intake and reducing sugary drinks. Watch the effect it has on your body, your skin, your sleep and your mood. A really simple tip – something I have done for years – is to fill or buy two 1.5-litre bottles in the morning and aim to have them finished by the end of the day. It's a very easy way of keeping track of how much water you're actually getting.

Alcohol: Let's face it – Irish people are both very attached to alcohol and not very clear about its wide-ranging effects. I see this all the time when I go through food diaries with new clients. They are often shocked, not only by the volume of alcohol they are consuming, but also to realize that alcohol…

- is laden with calories
- will dramatically increase your body-fat levels
- has a direct impact on your metabolism
- affects your mood in a negative way
- increases the chances of you eating high-sugar, low-nutrient foods in the days after consumption
- directly affects your health in lots of ways

The reality is that what you drink and how much you drink affects everything around you. We all know about the social impact of excessive drinking and the dangers of drink driving. But sticking solely to its effects on your weight, it's very easy to lose track of what you're drinking and it can derail your health plans quicker than pretty much anything else out there. Calories in alcohol are basically empty calories that are of little or no benefit to the body.

The table on the following page shows rough calorie counts for different drinks and what these calorie counts equate to in terms of food, and also how many calories you might be taking in from alcohol over the course of a year, depending on your weekly consumption.

I'm not going to be a killjoy and say never drink again. For most social drinkers, that won't happen. Indeed, I enjoy one or two bottles of organic cider a week myself. And alcohol can be good for you – obviously binge drinking is never healthy, but a glass or two of wine or cider or your tipple of choice will do you no harm whatsoever. It's a means of relaxation and can be part of a healthy, balanced lifestyle.

But instead of having a glass of wine, or two, every night, which has become so common, why not limit it to one night a week? And, of course, the better the

DRINK	AVERAGE CALORIES	SAME AS	CALORIES PER YEAR once a week	CALORIES PER YEAR five times a week	CALORIES PER YEAR ten times a week
WINE – bottle (750 ml)	684	Whopper burger	35,568	117,840	355,680
WINE – glass (175ml)	150	Bounty bar	7,800	39,000	78,000
CHAMPAGNE	90	Chocolate digestive biscuit	4,680	23,400	46,800
BEER (pint)	225	Slice of apple tart	11,700	58,500	117,000
CIDER (pint)	210	Mars bar	10,920	54,600	109,200
GUINNESS (pint)	210	5 Jaffa cakes	10,920	54,600	109,200
SPIRITS with mixers	110	Packet of crisps	5,720	28,600	57,200

quality of the product, the better it is for you. Aim to drink craft beers or ciders and decent wine (the quality of wines in supermarkets is very good now).

So, don't try to cut out drink altogether but create a balanced approach. Here are some simple tips that will help you get through those dinners and nights out as best you can. (You'll notice that a lot of these involve water. Because alcohol is a diuretic, it helps your body to excrete water before it can be absorbed – not only bad for you overall, but dehydration is a major cause of hangovers!)

Top tips for avoiding hangovers

- ☐ Never go out on an empty stomach. Have a low GI snack or light meal beforehand.

- ☐ Go for craft and organic products as much as possible.

- ☐ Order a glass of water with your drink and try to match your intake of alcohol and water.

- ☐ Aim for a glass of water in between drinks.

- ☐ Aim for a pint of water before bed (leave a full glass on your bedside table before you go out).

- ☐ Have a sachet of Dioralyte before bed – it will help rehydrate the body and, as alcohol gives your body a sugar rush, it will also help normalize your blood sugars.

- ☐ Always eat breakfast the next day, ideally a healthy one.

- ☐ Don't think you've blown it if you have a big night out – restrict yourself to one treat meal the next day and drink 3 litres of water. Soon you'll be back on track!

8 THE SEVEN-DAY KICK-START CHALLENGE

Enough of the theory! Here is a fast way to make use of the information I have given you so far to kick-start your diet. This is a seven-day challenge and here are my golden dozen – rules that are totally manageable and sure-fire ways of getting you to eat more healthily. A week of eating like this and you will be ready to keep up many, if not all, of these good habits.

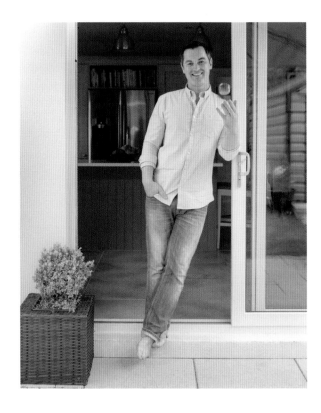

The Golden Dozen

1   At the beginning of the week, measure at least one of the three things I talked about in Chapter 2 (*see* page 20) – resting heart rate, waist or weight. Measure all three if you like.

2   Before you have breakfast, drink a glass of warm water with lemon slices or squeezed lemon juice.

3   Eat three meals and two snacks each day.

4   Switch from white foods to brown foods.

5   Have fruit every day, but no more than two pieces.

6   Reduce added sugars as much as you can – read labels.

7   Do not eat any diet, low-fat or sugar-free products.

8   Eat slowly and stop eating when you feel pleasantly full but not stuffed.

9   Drink 2 to 3 litres of water a day, with lemon or lime juice if you like.

10   Avoid fizzy drinks.

11   Have one treat meal (but don't go mad and try to include everything you missed all week in one big blow-out! Pick something you really love, eat it slowly, relish it and remind yourself that when you're in control and eating healthily most of the time you have leeway for occasional treats).

12   Whatever you measured at the start of the week, measure again.

Before you start, it's crucial to reduce temptation as much as you can. Get a box and place all the junk that's in your cupboards into it – all the sauces, biscuits and other junk that you now know you shouldn't be eating or drinking. Give the box away – to a neighbour or colleague – or even just throw it out. Plan for success, and this tip is one of the easiest ways to do it. If it's not there, you can't eat or drink it!

If you take this seven-day challenge, in that very short amount of time, you will start to see benefits, such as:

- more energy
- better digestion
- better sleep
- better mood
- less fluid retention
- a flatter stomach
- better skin
- better hair and nails

That is the good news. The bad news is that if you have a diet that is high in processed foods, caffeine or sugar, you may have some withdrawal symptoms. These are the main ones:

- low energy
- poor sleep
- poor mood
- bad skin
- headaches

Yes, I know these seem to contradict the first list – but they're temporary! If you get any of these, they will pass after a few days, so don't worry about it. Just stay focused, drink plenty of water and whatever you do, don't give up. By not giving up you will feel so good afterwards that it will be well worth it. (Obviously, if you have any serious symptoms that worry you, please consult your GP.)

Here is a simple chart we give to our clients when they sign up with us for personal training, which may guide you in terms of what you should be eating.

INCREASE	REDUCE	AVOID
water	milk – switch to semi-skimmed	fizzy drinks
grilled meats	white bread – switch to brown	fried foods
greens – broccoli, green beans, etc.	white rice – switch to brown	takeaways
all vegetables (except mashed potatoes)	white pasta – switch to brown	processed cereals
nuts	coffee/tea – reduce to 2 cups per day	cakes/pastries/ biscuits/buns
fish	alcohol (beer/wine/ spirits) – max. 4 glasses per week ('glass' means standard pub measures, not home measures i.e. half pint/425ml beer; 100ml wine; 35ml spirits)	pasteurized fruit juices
eggs		foods with 'diet' on the label
wholegrains		*But don't forget you can have a treat meal each week!*
natural yoghurt		
porridge		
fruit – max. 2 pieces per day	chocolate (less than 70% cocoa solids)	
brown foods		
natural foods	artificial butters – switch to real butter	
short-shelf-life foods		
herbal teas		
dark chocolate (70% or more cocoa solids)		

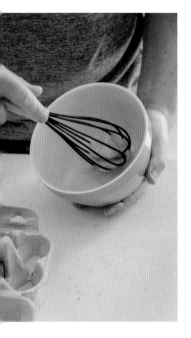

To make things even easier, here are examples of the types of meals you could choose from over the week (asterisks indicate that there are recipes later in the book). If you pick from these lists, you will be well on your way to improving your diet:

BREAKFAST

- Wholegrain toast
- Eggs: scrambled*/poached/boiled/baked*/ omelette*
- Homemade granola* or low-sugar branded one
- Freshly squeezed juices/ones with a short shelf life
- Homemade oat/fruit smoothie* if you're on the go
- Porridge*
- Overnight oats*

Whether you base breakfast on protein (e.g. eggs) or carbohydrates (e.g. porridge), make sure you have breakfast. It gets your metabolism fired up, decreases your chances of snacking during the day and gives you the fuel you need to get through your day. No matter how busy your day or how early you get up in the morning, it is the one meal you shouldn't skip.

LUNCH

- Salads with some form of protein*
- Brown rolls/bread/wraps*
- Soup*/brown bread*

DINNER

- Protein (e.g. chicken, chops, a piece of fish, bean dishes) with lots of vegetables*
- Brown pasta*
- Brown rice*
- Broths*

- Tomato-based rather than creamy sauces
- Stir fries* (fantastic and so quick to make)

A combination of protein and vegetables is the perfect meal. Filling up your plate with colourful vegetables and including a smaller proportion of rice/pasta/noodles/potatoes is a great way to make your dinner healthier. As well as being packed with minerals and vitamins, vegetables contain the best type of carbohydrates you can get and will fill you up. And they are great for gut health and digestion.

A final tip: if you're eating dinner late in the evening (say, after 8 pm), try to keep it light (or even plan to have a bigger lunch and a small evening meal).

SNACKS

- Soup* (but not ones laden with butter or cream or made with potatoes)
- Hummus* or guacamole with cucumber or carrot sticks
- Natural or Greek yoghurt (with some seeds and/or berries if you like)*
- Seeded Ryvita with smoked salmon
- Nuts (not covered in chocolate or yoghurt or salted)
- Seeds such as pumpkin, sunflower, flax, sesame
- Pear or apple with nut butter
- Fresh fruit with some nuts and seeds
- Pulled protein cooked the night before
- Poached or boiled eggs
- Homemade protein balls or granola bars
- Vegetable-based juice

If you're eating dinner late in the evening - say, after 8 pm - try to keep it light.

By making simple changes in what you eat and how you eat for just a week, you'll start to see the benefits to your body, your digestion, your mood and your overall health. I am confident that once you start, you will want to keep going – gradually feeling better, losing weight and becoming healthier.

9 WHAT TO EAT ON THE GO

Between work and holidays, we all travel more than ever before, and it probably provides the greatest challenge to maintaining a healthy diet, so let's take a look at what you can do to improve your food choices when you are travelling. When you pick up a product while in transit, ask yourself:

- Is it a real food or is it processed?
- Does it have a long or short shelf life?
- Does it have many or few ingredients?
- What has the least amount of sugar?
- Are there fruits or nuts available?
- Are you actually hungry or are you eating from habit or boredom?

If going on a flight, try to bring something from home (as long as it's not liquid, you should get it through security) or pick up something in the airport shops after security rather than eating what's served on the plane. Most airports now have a range of shops that offer healthy options. (Keep in mind that because of nut allergies some airlines do not permit passengers to bring nuts on flights. Also, unless you have already checked what's permitted and what's banned, you should dispose of foodstuffs before going through arrivals at your destination, as many countries have strict rules about what foods they allow in.)

Drink lots of fluids before, during and after any flights.

If you're on the road, keep this saying in mind: 'Don't refuel yourself where you refuel your car.' Most garages and motorway service stops in Ireland offer few healthy options. Apart from fruit and perhaps some nuts in their natural state, you'll struggle to find anything that isn't very calorific or sugary. Bring your own healthy snacks for the road.

When you're on holiday or away for work and eating out, the same rules apply as at home. If you order dishes that are in their most natural state, and have been treated as simply as possible, and if you keep your portions modest, you'll be on the right track. Of course, you will want to check out the local cuisine and specialities – just apply the treat rule on a slightly more generous basis. Keep your drinking and treat meals to a few times during the trip or holiday, rather than every meal every day.

And, of course, if you're in self-catering accommodation, all the suggestions I've made already about how to shop and cook apply. Indeed, you can make it an exciting opportunity to try healthy new foods in their natural habitat! I have a longer section on keeping healthy on holidays.

If you're on the road, keep this saying in mind: 'Don't refuel yourself where you refuel your car.' ... Bring your own healthy snacks for the road.

10 GET COOKING!

Having looked at food and the changes you need to make to lose weight and be healthier, it's now time to get cooking. I have to be honest and admit that my relationship with cooking is pretty average – you probably don't expect to hear that in a book where someone is sharing recipes! But that's all the more reason why I think you will find this section extremely user-friendly. When it comes to cooking, I'm very much the average Joe in my background and approach. So I believe that I have a grip on what most people need to know about making tasty food.

I grew up in the eighties and early nineties in a household of fairly standard home-cooked meals (roast chicken, spuds and veg; spag bol; chilli con carne; leg of lamb, etc.). However, my mum had a catering business and made health-food products from cottage cheese for many of the gyms in Dublin, so I grew up around that too – watching and helping out when I wasn't in school or at my dad's gym. This is how I learned the food basics and the tools that I now use.

When I went to college I forgot everything I knew! I had a small bedsit and, as with many a first-year student, the lads at the local takeaways became my new best friends. Though I played rugby and was getting more involved in the gym, the saying that you can't out-train a bad diet was definitely true in my case. I needed a wake-up call about how I was eating, and like a lot of people, it came via a photograph –

I could not deny the truth of what my bloated face was telling me. As well as that, I went hill walking in Wicklow one weekend and a member of our gym who was in his sixties put me to shame by beating me up Djouce Mountain by about 20 minutes. Shortly after, I bought a gas hob for the bedsit (not something most landlords would approve of, I guess!) and started cooking again – making my own meals, stir-fries mainly, and slowly developing a repertoire.

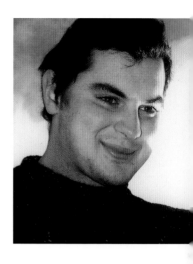

Fifteen years later, my relationship with food is what I consider normal – not over the top or complicated, just normal. As I recommend to you, I like to have the odd treat meal (my main weakness is pizza – really good pizza on a thin base!). From time to time, I end up turning to food when I get stressed, like so many people (that's if I haven't gone to the other extreme and gone mad exercising!). And I am increasing my knowledge of food and cooking all the time.

The average person is too busy to have to think about food, diet and weight constantly. Meals should be part of a balanced lifestyle. Healthy eating is about coming back to real food and learning some skills so you can cook it. (Speaking of skills, YouTube is a fantastic resource for the novice cook. It's full of demos on everything you'll need to do in the kitchen. Some of the best chefs, and chef instructors, in the world have videos up on everything from how to chop an onion to how to butcher a pig. And, of course, the internet is an almost infinite source of healthy recipe ideas. If you start sourcing recipes from US websites, add a set of measuring cups to the list below, as they measure everything in cups.)

Healthy eating is about coming back to real food and learning some skills so you can cook it.

As I said at the top, I am a basic cook, but I have learned what does and doesn't work. The recipes in the chapters that follow are some of my favourites to get you going. These are all things that I have developed over the years and have shared with clients too, so I have had plenty of feedback on them. I know

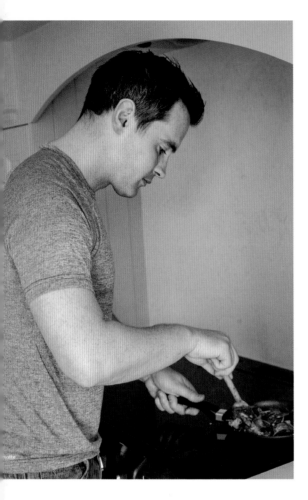

these are delicious, nutritious, reliable, quick and doable. They use ingredients you will find easily wherever you live. Trust me, if I can cook these then you certainly can too! And, of course, if you're an experienced cook these will be a doddle and you'll be able to add your own touches to make them more your own.

Before moving on to the recipes, here's a bit of housekeeping – a list of kit that will make preparing food far easier.

You may notice I don't include a food processor in this list (though I do mention one in the recipes that follow). I suggest that you see how you get on with this lot. After a while, you'll be able to judge how much time you would save by getting a food processor, what kind of attachments you would use, what size it should be and so on. As I do a lot of batch cooking, I use a food processor for convenience and I have plenty of cupboard space to store it. You might find you can get by quite easily without one – perhaps with the addition of a mini-chopper – and if you have a small kitchen, you won't want something sitting on the counter taking up a lot of space if you don't really need it.

Oven temperatures: All electric oven temperatures in the recipes are for a conventional oven. If you use a fan oven, simply reduce the temperature given by 20°C/35°F.

Key Kitchen Kit

- [ ] a set of kitchen knives (including a bread knife) and a knife sharpener
- [ ] large wooden or silicone spoons
- [ ] a range of silicone spatulas
- [ ] kitchen tongs
- [ ] a large slotted turner/fish slice
- [ ] a good pair of scissors or kitchen shears
- [ ] a box grater
- [ ] a couple of chopping boards (make sure you never use the same one for raw meat and other foods, at least not without first washing it thoroughly and drying with kitchen paper)
- [ ] a wok
- [ ] a large non-stick frying pan
- [ ] a set of stainless-steel heavy-bottomed saucepans, ideally with clear lids
- [ ] a large stockpot
- [ ] a measuring jug
- [ ] weighing scales
- [ ] measuring spoons
- [ ] a large strainer or colander
- [ ] a large sieve
- [ ] a stick blender

- [ ] a blender for smoothies (or a NutriBullet)
- [ ] a pepper mill
- [ ] a coffee grinder if you like to cook with spices – you can use it to grind them up
- [ ] a range of mixing bowls
- [ ] large Pyrex dishes – Pyrex dishes can go into the oven
- [ ] baking trays
- [ ] oven gloves – ideally non-slip waterproof silicone ones
- [ ] an apron – as much to get you 'in the zone' as to protect your clothes!
- [ ] a tin opener
- [ ] a vegetable peeler
- [ ] a corkscrew
- [ ] a George Foreman grill
- [ ] Tupperware containers
- [ ] tinfoil containers and lids for batch cooking (also, if you're cooking for one, save time by making up the whole recipe and then simply store the extra portions in the freezer)
- [ ] a book-stand for cookery books
- [ ] a journal to make notes and keep track of your favourite recipes

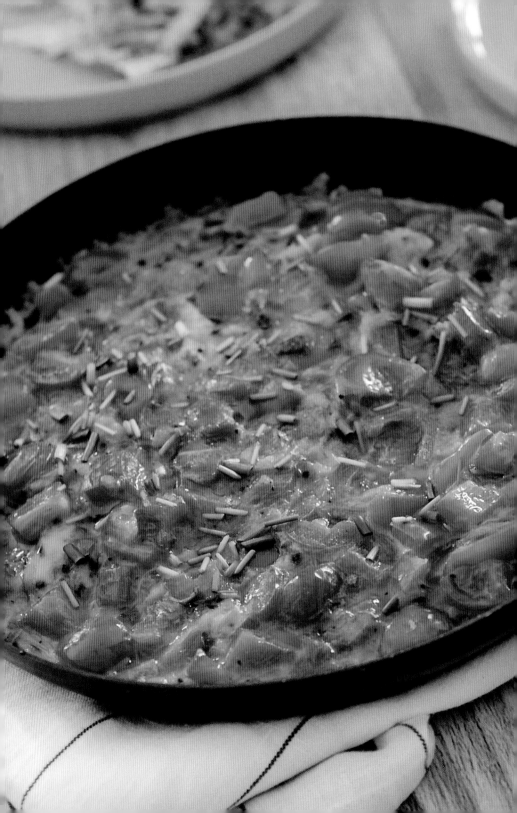

BREAKFAST RECIPES

11

KARL'S YUMMY GRANOLA

Granola is a quick and easy breakfast option and so simple to make. Most off-the-shelf granolas are really high in sugar and additives, so why not make your own?

PREP TIME 5 to 10 minutes
COOKING TIME 25 minutes
SERVES 10

400g jumbo oats
75g mixed seeds
75g honey
75g coconut oil
75g mixed nuts
75g desiccated coconut
50g dried apricots, finely
   chopped

COCONUT OIL
Even though it's solid at room temperature, coconut oil is actually a liquid and you'll notice the measurement on the jar is in ml. To translate the gram measurement to ml, add 10 per cent. In other words, 100g of coconut oil is 110ml. The measurement in this recipe – 75g – is 82ml (but you can round to 80 or 85; it doesn't have to be exact). If you come across the ml measurement for coconut oil in a recipe and want to convert to grams, then just deduct 10 per cent – so 100ml is about 90g.

1 Preheat the oven to 180°C/350°F/gas mark 4 and line a large baking tray with greaseproof paper. This ensures that the ingredients don't stick to the tray.

2 Mix the oats and seeds with the honey and coconut oil, spread out evenly on the baking tray and place in the middle of the oven.

3 After 10 minutes, remove from the oven and sprinkle over the mixed nuts, being careful not to touch any of the hot surfaces. Using a large spoon or spatula, stir the mixture on the tray. Return to the oven and bake for another 10 minutes.

4 Then, in the same way, remove from the oven again, add the desiccated coconut, stir again, and return to the oven to bake for another 5 minutes.

5 Allow to cool (for about 30 minutes) and then add the chopped apricots.

6 Keeps very well in a sealed container for three to four weeks. Granola can be used in lots of ways: as a cereal with milk (dairy, nut, soya), sprinkled on yoghurt with berries or dry as a snack (but don't go mad – while it's a lot healthier than a bag of crisps, it's still high in calories! A normal serving would be ½ a small mug, which contains approximately 200 calories).

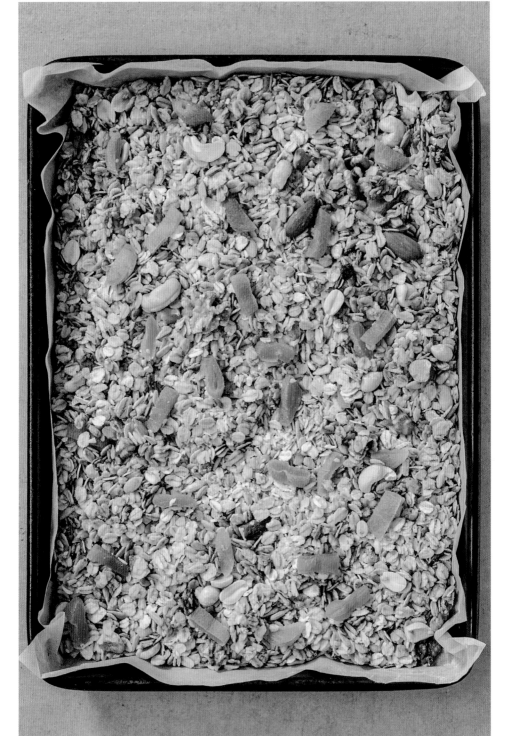

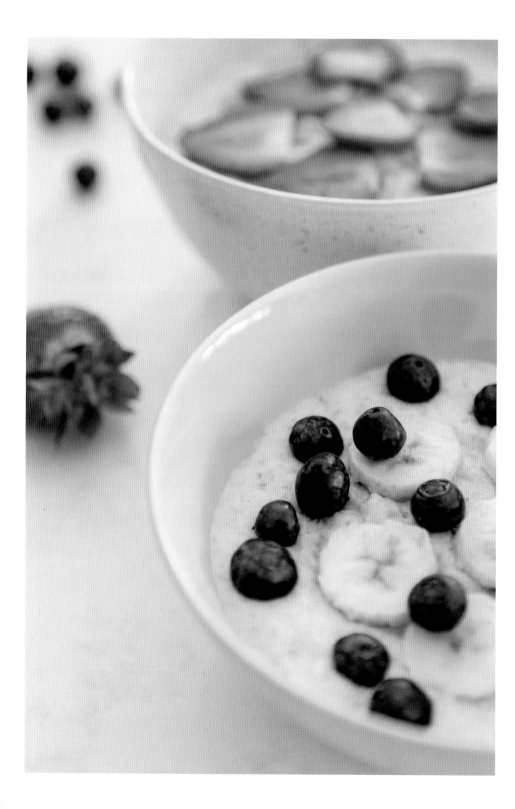

PORRIDGE, TWO WAYS

I am porridge's biggest fan! It's delicious, full of slow-release energy, super-healthy and cheap too. My simple porridge trick is to soak the oats overnight – they not only cook more quickly in the morning, but the porridge tastes even better too. You can put on a variety of toppings – I give you two suggestions here, chia and strawberries or banana and blueberries.

1 Place the porridge oats, water and milk in a small saucepan over a high heat. Bring to the boil.

2 Reduce the heat to medium, stir and simmer for 4 to 5 minutes, stirring occasionally, until the oats have absorbed the fluid and it has thickened. Now that the oats are cooked, you can change the consistency of the porridge by adding more milk and stirring it in. Personally, I love thick porridge, but you can adjust the consistency to your liking really easily.

3 If you decide to soak the oats overnight, use 160ml of water or milk. Heat through gently in the morning – there is no need to boil. Again, if the consistency is too thick for you, add some more liquid to loosen.

4 Divide between two bowls and sprinkle with the chia seeds and strawberries or the sliced bananas and blueberries.

PREP AND COOKING TIME 10 minutes
SERVES 2

75g jumbo porridge oats
160ml water
160ml milk (dairy, nut, soya – whichever you prefer)

VERSION 1
2 tsp chia seeds
8 to 10 fresh strawberries, hulled and sliced

VERSION 2
1 banana, sliced
125g punnet fresh blueberries

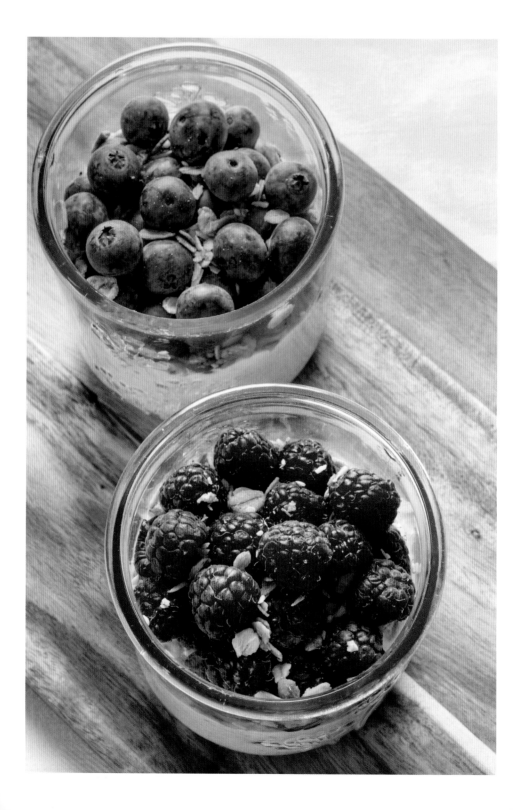

SUPER-SIMPLE OVERNIGHT OATS

This is my version of one of the trendiest breakfast options around. Delicious, quick to make and loaded with slow-release carbohydrates, this is the perfect go-to option if you are in a hurry in the morning.

1 Wash four glass jars (ones with capacity of about 200ml) and their lids in hot water and dry thoroughly.

2 Combine the yoghurt, coconut milk and vanilla extract in a small bowl.

3 Layer the oats, chia seeds and blueberries (or raspberries) in the four jars.

4 Divide the yoghurt mixture evenly between the four jars, pouring it over the dry ingredients.

5 Sprinkle a few fresh blueberries or raspberries on top of the mixture in each jar and screw on the lids.

6 Chill overnight in the fridge. Just before eating, sprinkle 1 tablespoon of the granola into each jar.

7 These overnight oats will keep for up to three days in the fridge, so you can eat whenever it suits you!

8 If this mixture makes the oats too thick for you, just add more milk to get them to your desired consistency. And, of course, the longer you leave the oats, the more of the liquid they will absorb, so add more milk to loosen if needed. You'll quickly discover how to make your overnight oats just right for you!

PREP TIME 5 minutes
SERVES 4

200ml Greek yoghurt
200ml coconut milk
   (see last note below)
1 tsp vanilla extract
200g jumbo porridge oats
8 tbsp chia seeds
125g blueberries or
   raspberries, plus extra
   for sprinkling
4 tbsp granola (hopefully
   homemade using the
   recipe on page 72; if
   not, please use a
   low-sugar version)

SCRAMBLED EGGS WITH CHORIZO AND SPINACH

This recipe has everything! Eggs are full of protein, spinach is an amazing source of vitamins and minerals, and the chorizo will add some healthy fat, as well as making this recipe super-tasty. I add a generous amount of black pepper to give it a nice kick. As the chorizo is naturally salty, you probably won't need any additional salt to season.

PREP TIME 5 minutes
COOKING TIME 5 minutes
SERVES 1

75g chorizo, diced into
1cm chunks
2 large free-range eggs,
beaten
a large handful of baby
spinach leaves
freshly ground black
pepper

1 Using a non-stick pan, fry the chorizo over a low heat. You won't need to add any fat as the fat in the chorizo will melt down and help to fry the lean part. Fry until the chorizo pieces are crisp.

2 Remove the pan from the heat. Push the cooked chorizo to one side of the pan and, using a few sheets of kitchen paper, blot away the fat that's rendered out and put it in the bin (you don't want to pour it down the sink as it may solidify and block your drain!).

3 Add the beaten eggs and allow to cook, agitating and stirring them a little, before adding the spinach and the chorizo. I like my scrambled eggs well cooked, so I make sure they're solid before adding the spinach. If you like them softer, you can add the spinach while they're still a little runny.

4 Stir the mixture until the spinach softens and wilts – this will happen very quickly, in a minute or two. Season with black pepper.

5 These scrambled eggs are delicious on their own or with a slice of wholemeal or sourdough bread.

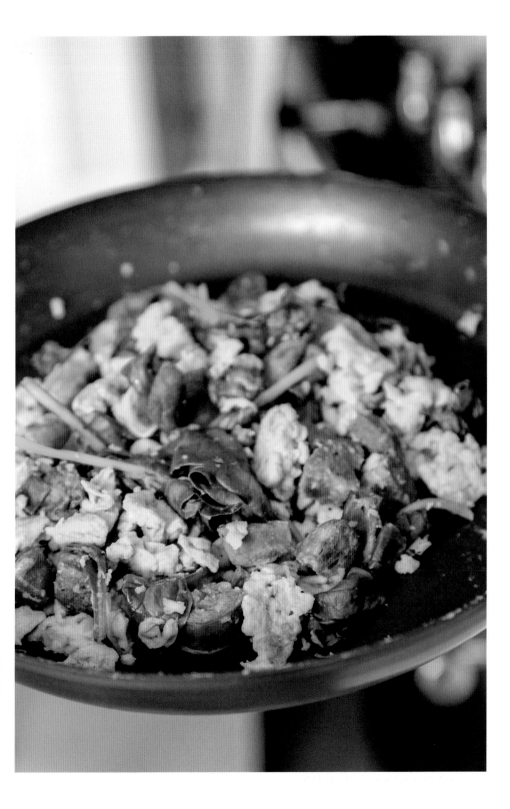

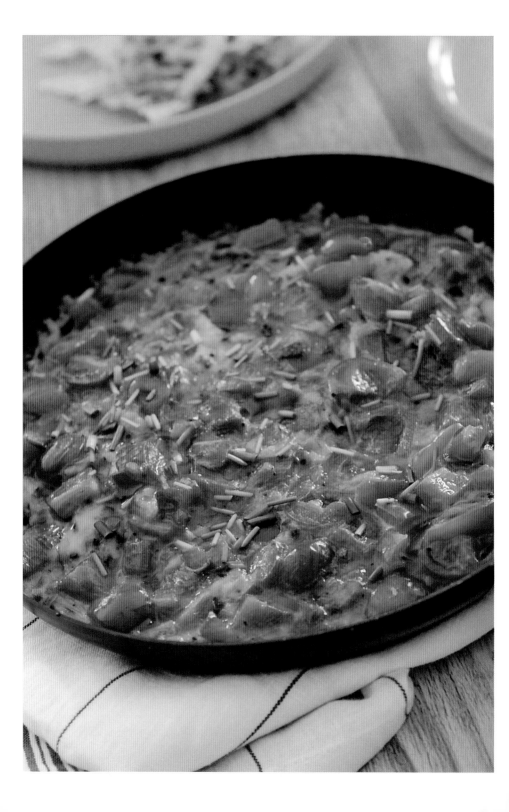

RAINBOW OMELETTE

Omelettes are a great way of getting a healthy meal into your day. They are quick to make and you can fill them with whatever you want. Ideally, make them full of colour, as colourful vegetables are full of minerals, vitamins and antioxidants. Omelettes are also a great source of protein. This is one of my favourites.

1 Put a non-stick pan on to a medium heat and pour the oil into the pan.

2 When the oil is hot, put the chopped peppers and onion into the pan and leave to cook, stirring occasionally. Add in the tomatoes when the other vegetables are already nice and soft.

3 Meanwhile, crack the eggs into a bowl, add seasoning to taste and beat lightly with a fork.

4 When the tomatoes have broken down slightly, add the beaten eggs to the pan and stir through lightly.

5 Allow to cook for about 6 minutes or until the eggs have set to your taste.

6 You can adapt this simple omelette recipe to incorporate your favourite veg for a healthy breakfast any time of year. It's good for lunch or a quick supper too, and you can bump up the nutritional value if you add a little salad on the side!

PREP TIME 5 minutes
COOKING TIME 5 minutes
SERVES 2

1 tbsp rapeseed oil
1 red pepper, chopped
1 jalapeño pepper, finely chopped (if you like hot food, you can add more than one!)
½ small red onion, peeled and finely chopped
6 cherry tomatoes, quartered
4 eggs
sea salt and freshly ground black pepper

BAKED EGGS WITH TABASCO AND TOMATO SALSA

Baked eggs are a really simple twist for breakfast; they are quick to cook, full of protein and a delicious way to start off your day. Don't be put off by the baking – it couldn't be easier!

PREP TIME 2 minutes
COOKING TIME 15 minutes
SERVES 1

½ tsp rapeseed oil
2 eggs
1 tomato, chopped
1 spring onion, chopped
1 tsp chopped coriander
a dash of Tabasco
sea salt and freshly
   ground black pepper

1 Preheat the oven to 180°C/350°F/gas mark 4. Oil a small ovenproof dish using the rapeseed oil.

2 Break the eggs into the dish. Put into the centre of the preheated oven and bake for 12 to 15 minutes, until the egg whites are just set.

3 Meanwhile, make the salsa by mixing the chopped tomato, spring onion and coriander with the Tabasco in a small bowl. Season to taste.

4 Remove the eggs from the oven. You can serve them in the dish they've been cooked in. Delicious with the lovely fresh salsa and some toast!

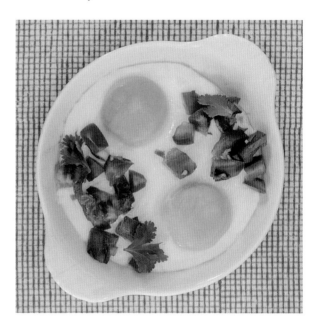

AVOCADO TOASTIE

Avocado toasties have become a breakfast favourite – and for very good reason! They're quick, easy, filling and super-nutritious. This is a great go-to breakfast if you have a busy morning ahead. My take on the avocado toastie has a hint of hot sauce because I like a bit of heat in my food.

1 Put the bread on to toast.

2 Using a fork, mash the avocado flesh in a bowl with the olive oil, the lime juice and a couple of splashes of the Tabasco or hot sauce. If you like spicy foods, you can add more.

3 Spread the avocado mix on the toast while it's still hot.

4 To make this a weekend brunch dish, you could add a poached egg on top of one of your toasties!

PREP TIME 5 minutes
SERVES 1

2 slices of wholegrain bread
1 medium-sized avocado, peeled, halved and stoned
1 tsp olive oil
juice of ½ small lime
a few dashes of Tabasco or hot sauce

AVOCADOS

Avocados are delicious but can be tricky to buy, often being either rock hard or starting to go off – and it's not always obvious which it is from the outside. When buying, make sure the skin is evenly coloured with no darker patches. Very gently squeeze them to see if there's a little give. If there is too much give, chances are that the avocado is starting to go off. If avocados are hard, you can still buy them. Just place them in a brown paper bag with a ripening banana, leave on a shelf in the kitchen and they will be perfectly ripe in a couple of days! If you are using just half the avocado, cut through the length around the stone, which will remain with one side or the other. Use the side without the stone and keep the half with the stone in the fridge.

SUPER-QUICK AND NUTRITIOUS SMOOTHIES

Sometimes there is very little time in the morning to prepare breakfast, so popping a few lovely fresh ingredients into a blender is a great way of getting a filling nutritional hit in very little time. In fact, the first smoothie here is a perfect option for preparing the night before and grabbing from the fridge as you run out the door!

PREP TIME 6 minutes
SERVES 1

200g pineapple, peeled and roughly chopped
☐ medium red pepper
½ small avocado, peeled, halved and stoned
a handful of spinach leaves, washed
a handful of kale leaves, with stalks, washed
juice of 1 large juicy orange
juice of ½ lime
1 tbsp water, to loosen mixture (optional)

TANGY GREEN SMOOTHIE

1 Put all the dry ingredients into a blender or NutriBullet. Pour the juices on top.

2 Cover and blitz for about 20 seconds until everything is well combined. You will end up with a vibrant green smoothie that tastes lovely and fruity!

3 You can substitute any fruit that you have in your fridge for the pineapple. You can also add the tablespoon of water, or more if needed, to loosen the consistency if you find it is too thick.

4 This smoothie will usually last for two days in the fridge.

CREAMY APPLE AND PEAR SMOOTHIE

PREP TIME 5 minutes
SERVES 1

1 Throw the apple and pear whole into your blender or NutriBullet (remove stalks but there's no need to remove the core – it's all good fibrous stuff!). Then put in the rest of the dry ingredients.

2 Pour over the milk and drizzle with the honey.

3 Cover and blitz for about 20 seconds until everything is well combined.

4 This smoothie will usually last for two days in the fridge.

1 small, unpeeled apple
1 unpeeled pear, ideally soft
a handful of shredded kale, with stalks
2 tbsp jumbo porridge oats
3 thin slices of fresh ginger, diced
300ml milk (dairy, nut or soya)
½ tsp honey

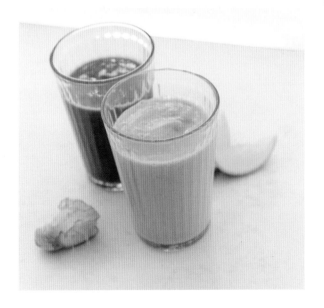

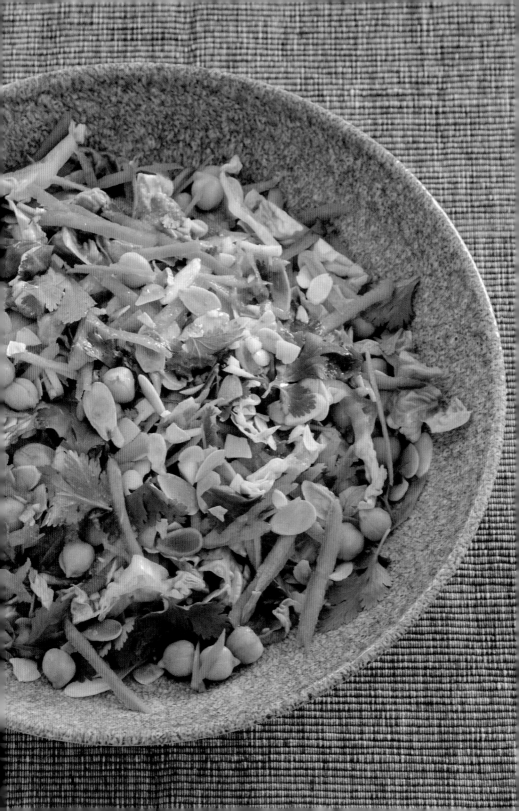

LUNCH RECIPES

12

EVERYDAY VEGETABLE SOUP

THAI CHICKEN SOUP

CHICKEN, VEGETABLE AND NOODLE SOUP

SPINACH AND GOAT'S CHEESE WRAP

PRAWN KEBABS WITH MIXED LEAVES

BAKED SWEET POTATO WITH ROASTED VEGETABLES

GO-TO SPICY SALAD

MOROCCAN CHICKPEA AND CARROT SALAD

TWO SIMPLE STOCK RECIPES

EVERYDAY VEGETABLE SOUP

Soup is one of my favourite things to make – so simple, so delicious and full of nutrients. A great filling meal, especially if you get home late at night as I often do!

PREP TIME 10 minutes
COOKING TIME 40 minutes
SERVES 4

1 tsp rapeseed oil
1 large onion, peeled and finely chopped
2 cloves of garlic, peeled and finely chopped
2 large carrots, scrubbed and thinly sliced (no need to peel)
2 medium sweet potatoes, peeled and cut into 1 to 2cm cubes
1 litre vegetable stock (use 2 vegetable stock cubes)
1 red pepper, roughly sliced
1 yellow pepper, roughly sliced
1 x 400g tin white beans, drained and rinsed
½ tsp dried basil
½ tsp dried oregano
2 dried bay leaves
1 tbsp soy sauce (optional)
½ medium head of broccoli – florets only

1 Heat the oil in a large saucepan over a medium heat and add the onion. Fry for two minutes, then reduce the heat and allow the onion to soften, stirring occasionally. If it starts to stick, add a tablespoon of water. It will be soft and golden in about 10 minutes.

2 Add the chopped garlic, carrots and sweet potatoes and the stock. Increase the heat to high and bring to the boil. Once the mixture has boiled, reduce the heat to low and simmer for about 10 minutes until the carrots and sweet potatoes are slightly tender (stick a fork in a piece to test this).

3 Add all the remaining ingredients except the broccoli and continue to simmer until the vegetables are soft – about 10 to 15 minutes.

4 Add the broccoli and simmer for 5 more minutes.

5 You can use a stick blender to whizz the soup together in the pan or let it cool slightly and pour into a liquidizer.

6 Once it's cool enough to taste, check for seasoning (when it's really hot, you won't be able to taste accurately). If you use stock cubes, you may not need to add salt as most stock cubes are a little salty.

7 Serve with a dollop of Greek yoghurt on top if you like.

8 Once you're happy making this soup, you can start to experiment with different combinations of veg that you like, or that are in season and cheap. You could, for instance, drop the carrot and sweet potato and add more broccoli to make that the hero of the soup. Just simmer until the broccoli is tender but still nice and green.

9 You can freeze this soup, so you may want to make more than you need and have a healthy option on standby for when you're pressed for time.

EXTRAS
a dollop of Greek yoghurt, to serve (optional)
sea salt (optional) and freshly ground black pepper

STOCK CUBES
It's best if you can use organic stock cubes, as they will have a better flavour and fewer additives. Most supermarkets have them. If not, you can get them in any health-food shop. It is very quick and easy to make your own vegetable stock too – see the recipes on page 100.

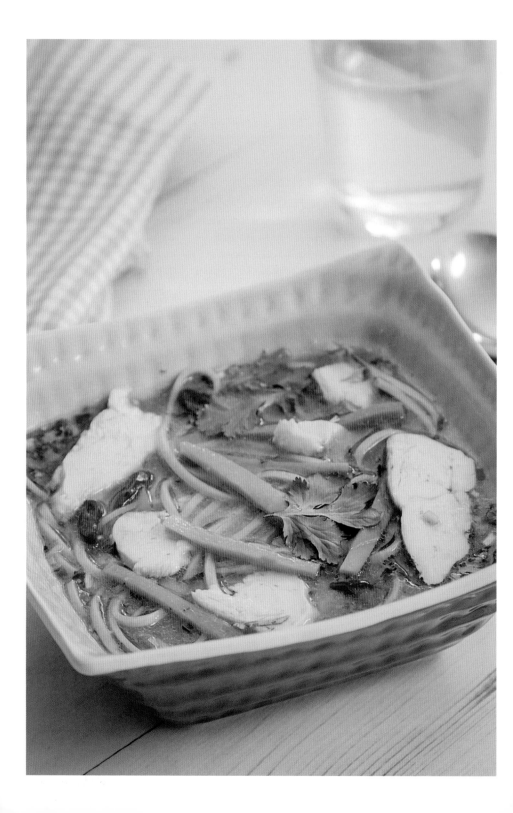

THAI CHICKEN SOUP

Between the chicken, the lovely fragrant Thai flavours and the filling noodles, you're getting a lot of great nutrients here in one warming, delicious bowl that feels like a treat.

1 Heat the oil in a large saucepan over a medium heat. Add the spring onions, garlic and ginger and cook for about 4 minutes, stirring frequently, until softened.

2 Add the carrots and chilli and cook for a further 2 minutes.

3 Add the curry paste, stock, lemongrass and a tablespoon of fish sauce and bring the mixture to the boil. Add the red pepper and noodles, then reduce the heat and simmer for a further 2 to 3 minutes.

4 Add the chicken and simmer for another 2 to 3 minutes, until the noodles are fully cooked (they should still have a tiny bite to them and not be soggy) and the chicken is heated through.

5 Add a tablespoon of lime juice and the chopped coriander and taste. Add more lime juice (for a more fragrant flavour) and/or more fish sauce (for a deeper, saltier flavour) if you like.

PREP TIME 10 minutes
COOKING TIME 15 minutes
SERVES 2

1 tbsp rapeseed oil
1 bunch of spring onions, thinly sliced
1 large clove of garlic, peeled and finely chopped
2cm piece of fresh ginger, peeled and finely chopped
2 carrots, peeled and finely chopped
1 red chilli, deseeded (if you prefer less heat) and thinly sliced
1 tbsp Thai green curry paste
650ml chicken stock
1 stick of lemongrass, crushed
1 tbsp fish sauce, plus extra to taste
1 red pepper, sliced lengthways
50g wholewheat noodles
1 cooked chicken breast, shredded or finely diced
1 tbsp lime juice, plus extra to taste
a handful of fresh coriander, chopped

CHICKEN, VEGETABLE AND NOODLE SOUP

This is one of my favourite filling soups, as it just feels so warm and nourishing – when you eat it, you'll love it!

PREP TIME 10 minutes
COOKING TIME 15 to 20 minutes
SERVES 4

1 tbsp rapeseed oil
1 red chilli, deseeded
(if you prefer less heat)
and finely chopped
2cm piece of fresh ginger,
peeled and finely
chopped
1 clove of garlic, peeled
and finely chopped
3 large chicken breasts
(400 to 450g), thinly
sliced into strips
1 large head of broccoli,
cut into small florets
125g mushrooms, thinly
sliced
1 litre vegetable stock
(use 2 vegetable stock
cubes, or use
homemade – see recipe
on page 100)
200g wholewheat noodles
(4 nests)
2 tbsp soy sauce
a handful of fresh
coriander, chopped
juice of 1 lime

1 Heat the oil in a large saucepan over a medium heat. Add the chilli, ginger and garlic and cook for about a minute, stirring occasionally.

2 Add the chicken strips and fry in the saucepan over a medium heat, stirring frequently, until the chicken is cooked – about 3 minutes.

3 Add the broccoli, mushrooms, stock, noodles and soy sauce. Bring to the boil and then reduce the heat and simmer for 4 to 5 minutes until the broccoli is tender and the noodles are cooked.

4 To finish, add the coriander and lime juice and stir through.

SPINACH AND GOAT'S CHEESE WRAP

I've really got into using goat's cheese over the last few years. It is really delicious and delivers a huge flavour hit in a relatively small quantity. We are especially lucky to have so many great suppliers in Ireland.

1 Make a bed of spinach leaves on the wrap and sprinkle the grated carrot on top.

2 Use as much of the onion as you like, depending on taste (and if you're going to be in meetings in the afternoon!).

3 Crumble the goat's cheese finely on top and wrap or roll tightly.

PREP TIME 5 minutes
SERVES 1

a handful of baby spinach
    leaves, washed and
    dried
1 wholewheat wrap
1 small carrot, peeled and
    finely grated
¼ to ½ small red onion,
    very finely sliced
30g goat's cheese

PRAWN KEBABS WITH MIXED LEAVES

One of the easiest recipes in the book – delicious and super-healthy too. Once you master this kebab, you can use this method with other combos (chicken, beef, meaty fish and halloumi all work well) and you'll never be without a simple, quick, flavoursome lunch or light dinner.

PREP TIME 5 minutes
COOKING TIME 15 minutes
SERVES 2

juice of 1 lemon
½ tsp smoked paprika
1 clove of garlic, peeled and finely chopped
freshly ground black pepper
200g jumbo prawns
1 red onion, peeled and cut into chunks about the same size as the prawns
1 red pepper, cut into chunks about the same size as the prawns
1 pack of wooden kebab skewers, soaked in water for at least half an hour before cooking (this stops them burning)

1 Mix the lemon juice, paprika, garlic and black pepper (to taste) together in a bowl to make a marinade for the prawns.

2 Add the prawns to the bowl and coat thoroughly with the marinade. Leave in the fridge for at least 15 minutes. (If you have time, you can leave the prawns marinating for longer, but no more than a few hours.)

3 When you are ready to prepare the kebabs, take the skewers and thread with alternating prawns and pieces of onion and red pepper. Have each piece touching but not crammed together on the skewer. Leave a couple of centimetres bare at each end of the skewer. Brush each kebab with some of the marinade.

4 Heat the grill to medium and cook the kebabs for 15 minutes, turning occasionally, until they're golden and cooked through.

5 Serve with a side salad.

6 Once you have mastered this kebab, the sky is the limit in terms of what you can put on a skewer!

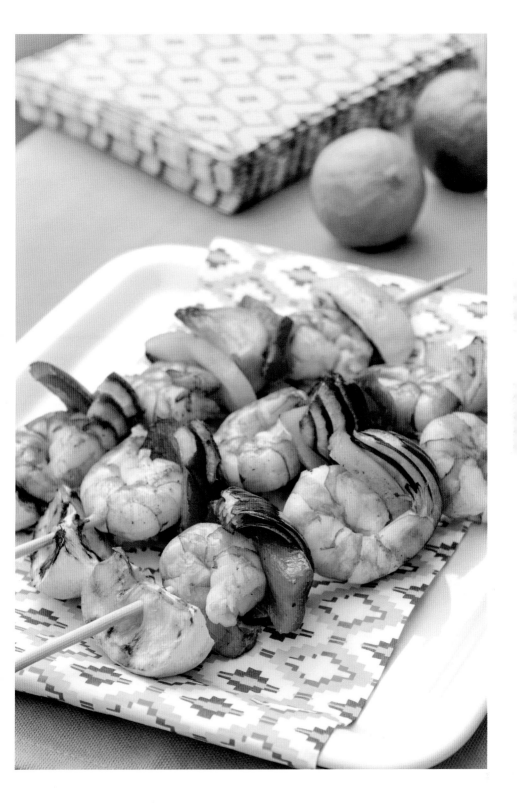

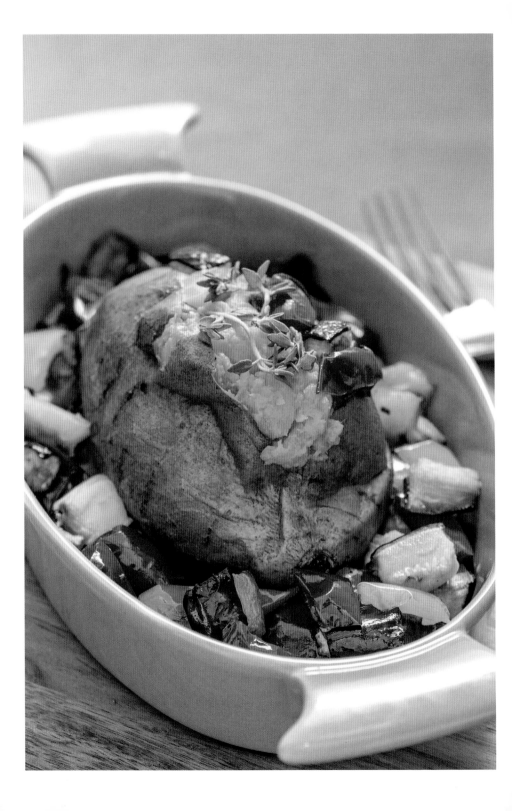

BAKED SWEET POTATO WITH ROASTED VEGETABLES

Sweet potato has never been more popular and it makes a great lunch dish, either hot or cold. Remember, you can eat the skin too – it's full of nutrients.

1 Preheat the oven to 180°C/350°F/gas mark 4.

2 Pierce the skins of the sweet potatoes, place in the middle of the preheated oven on one of the racks and bake for 1 hour.

3 Put the chopped pepper, courgette and aubergine into a roasting tray. Scatter the herbs on top and drizzle with the oil. Mix the veg to coat with the oil and spread out in a single layer on the tray. Put into the oven when the potatoes have been baking for 40 minutes (you can just nudge the potatoes to one side or put them on a higher or lower oven rack).

4 Check the sweet potatoes after an hour. They should be cooked through when you pierce them with a skewer or thin knife blade. The other veg should also be roasted.

5 Make a long cut or cross in the top of each potato, prise them open and pile the roasted veg on top.

PREP TIME 10 minutes
COOKING TIME 1 hour
SERVES 1

2 small sweet potatoes, scrubbed
1 red or yellow pepper, roughly chopped
1 courgette, sliced into 2cm chunks
½ aubergine, cut into 2cm cubes
small pinch of rosemary or thyme (dried or fresh, and finely chopped; you'll need less of the fresh herb)
1 to 2 tsp rapeseed oil

GO-TO SPICY SALAD

I love dishes with a bit of heat – always have! – so the salad dressing in this recipe has a bit of a kick to it. It's a really simple salad that you can make up with whatever is in season. And you can add a protein of your choice to beef it up (so to speak!). Protein is essential for the growth and repair of your muscles and crucial for your body.

PREP TIME 10 minutes
SERVES 2

FOR THE SALAD
1 small head of baby gem lettuce, torn
1 medium carrot, peeled and finely grated
1 beetroot (vacuum-packed, not pickled), cut into large dice
1 small red pepper, finely diced
1 cucumber, deseeded and diced
12 cherry tomatoes, halved
½ ripe avocado, peeled, halved, stoned and chopped
a handful of sugarsnap peas, sliced lengthways
2 spring onions, finely sliced
¼ to ½ red onion, peeled and finely sliced
¼ small red cabbage, finely shredded
¼ small head of broccoli, florets only

ADD ONE OF THE FOLLOWING
2 x 160g tins tuna, drained
2 cooked chicken breasts, chopped
6 cooked turkey slices, chopped (quantity based on meat sliced off the breast, not processed turkey slices)
1 x 400g tin chickpeas, drained and rinsed
1 x 400g tin butter beans, drained and rinsed

FOR THE DRESSING
juice of 2 limes
2 tsp soy sauce
a few drops of Tabasco
2 tsp sesame oil
sea salt and freshly ground black pepper, to taste

1 Mix your salad ingredients in a large bowl in whatever order you like – couldn't be simpler. If you're making the salad in advance, it's best to only cut and chop the avocado just before you're ready to eat the salad, as it quickly turns brown when exposed to the air. Also, if you're sensitive to raw onion, you can reduce or eliminate the red onion.

2 Mix the dressing ingredients in a small bowl with a fork or spoon. Keep in a little bottle or jar if you're not serving straight away. Give the dressing a good shake before pouring over your salad.

MOROCCAN CHICKPEA AND CARROT SALAD

A great salad, full of colour, that is quick to make and seriously filling too!

1 In a large bowl, mix the chickpeas, carrots, coriander or mint, flaked almonds and lettuce.

2 To make the dressing, mix the cumin, lemon juice, olive oil and garlic, and add the Tabasco if using.

3 Dress the salad and serve immediately.

PREP TIME 10 minutes
SERVES 2

FOR THE SALAD
1 x 200g tin chickpeas, drained and rinsed
2 carrots, peeled and chopped into matchstick pieces or shredded
a handful of fresh coriander or mint, finely chopped
1 tbsp flaked almonds, toasted
1 small head of baby gem lettuce, finely shredded

FOR THE DRESSING
½ tsp ground cumin
juice of ½ lemon
1 tbsp olive oil
½ clove of garlic, peeled and crushed
a dash of Tabasco (optional)

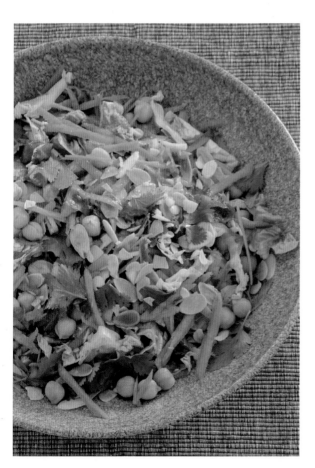

TWO SIMPLE STOCK RECIPES

It is unbelievably easy to make your own stock, and incredibly satisfying too! It's something I got into relatively recently. I do a big batch every few weeks and freeze it in smaller 500ml containers, so I always have a base for making my own soups. It's one of the few things I do that makes me feel properly cheffy in the kitchen!

1 tbsp rapeseed oil
2 onions, peeled and
   chopped
3 carrots, unpeeled,
   scrubbed and chopped
3 sticks of celery,
   chopped
3 cloves of garlic, peeled
   and chopped (optional)
2 litres water
2 bay leaves
a few sprigs of fresh
   thyme
a few sprigs of fresh
   parsley
sea salt and freshly
   ground black pepper

VEGETABLE STOCK

1 Heat the oil in a large saucepan and add the onions, carrots, celery and garlic (if using) and fry over a medium heat for 5 to 10 minutes or until they're slightly softened.

2 Add the 2 litres of water, the bay leaves and the thyme and parsley. Bring to the boil and then reduce the heat and simmer on low for 45 to 50 minutes. Season to taste, then strain through a sieve and leave to cool.

3 You can store the stock in the freezer in 500ml quantities.

BEEF STOCK

1 Preheat the oven to 200°C/400°F/gas mark 6.

2 Rub the oil over the bones and chopped up vegetables and place in a large roasting tin. Roast the bones, onions, carrots and celery for about 45 minutes.

3 Remove from the oven and put the roasted bones and vegetables into a large saucepan over a high heat with the bay leaf, thyme and parsley and the 3 litres of water and season to taste. Bring to the boil and then reduce the heat, simmering gently on a low heat for 5 to 6 hours. Skim any scum off the surface a few times during the first hour.

4 Use a slotted spoon to remove the bones and vegetables (you can bin them). Strain the liquid into a large container through a fine sieve and leave to cool. Scrape off any fat that solidifies on top and bin it (don't put it down the sink as it will block your pipes!).

5 You can store the stock in the freezer in 500ml quantities.

1.5kg beef bones (chopped up, the butcher can do this for you if you don't have a cleaver)
2 tbsp rapeseed oil
2 onions, peeled and chopped
2 to 3 carrots, unpeeled, scrubbed and chopped
3 sticks of celery, chopped
1 bay leaf
a sprig of fresh thyme
a sprig of fresh parsley
3 litres water
sea salt and freshly ground black pepper, to taste

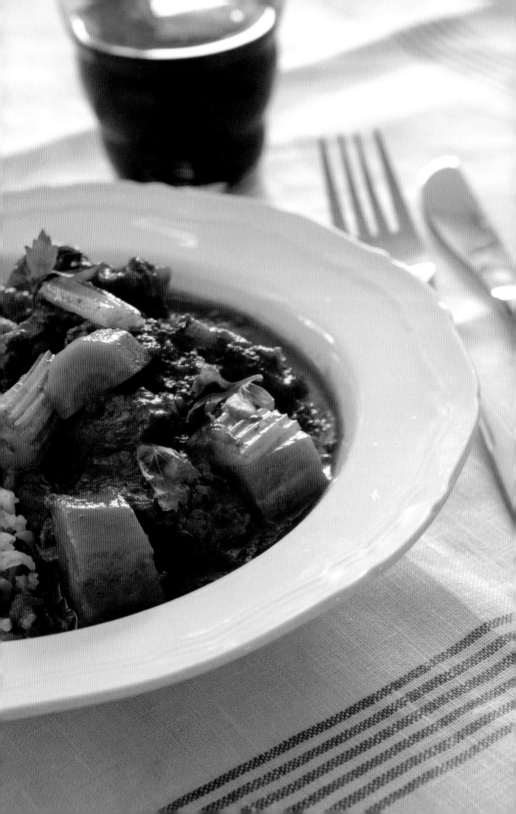

DINNER RECIPES

13

SUPER-QUICK CHICKEN AND VEGETABLE STIR-FRY

SUPERFOOD SALAD

KARL'S CREAMY CHICKEN AND SWEET POTATO TREAT

CHILLI CHICKEN PASTA

CHICKEN AND RED LENTIL CURRY

CRISPY CHICKEN GOUJONS

TURKEY BURGERS

LEAN AND JUICY MINCE

BAKED HAKE WITH SWEET POTATO

BAKED SALMON WITH MEDITERRANEAN VEGETABLES

HEALTHY ROAST VEGETABLE LASAGNE

A HEARTY HOTPOT

BEEF AND GUINNESS STEW

SUPER-QUICK CHICKEN AND VEGETABLE STIR-FRY

Stir-fries were one of the first dishes I cooked when I became conscious of eating more healthily. My cooking skills were fairly basic – to say the least! – but I could still rustle up a tasty dinner. Stir-fries are quick and simple to prepare and super-healthy. What's not to love?

PREP TIME 10 minutes
COOKING TIME 10 to 15 minutes
SERVES 2

2 tsp rapeseed oil
2 chicken fillets (125g each), sliced crossways into 1cm-thick strips
1 medium red onion, peeled and thinly sliced
1 medium red pepper, thinly sliced
200g mushrooms, thinly sliced
2 large handfuls of baby spinach (approx. 50g)
3 spring onions, sliced into 1cm pieces
1 clove of garlic, peeled and crushed
1 tbsp soy sauce
½ tsp sesame oil
1 tsp chopped coriander

1 Put the oil in a non-stick wok or large non-stick frying pan and heat on high until the oil is hot.

2 Add the chicken and cook on a high heat for 2 minutes, stirring continuously with a wooden or silicone spoon or spatula.

3 Reduce the heat to medium and add the sliced onion, pepper and mushrooms and cook for 3 minutes, stirring continuously, until the onion and pepper have lost their crispness and started to soften. Cook for a minute or two longer to soften further, adding a few drops of water if the pan is starting to dry out.

4 Add the spinach, spring onions and garlic, mix well and cook for a further 2 minutes, stirring occasionally.

5 Add the soy sauce and sesame oil and stir through.

6 Scatter the chopped coriander on top and you're ready to serve, either on its own or with brown rice or noodles.

7 One of the beauties of stir-fries is that you can add absolutely anything! This recipe will work just as well with thinly sliced beef, prawns or even tofu, and is just as quick to cook!

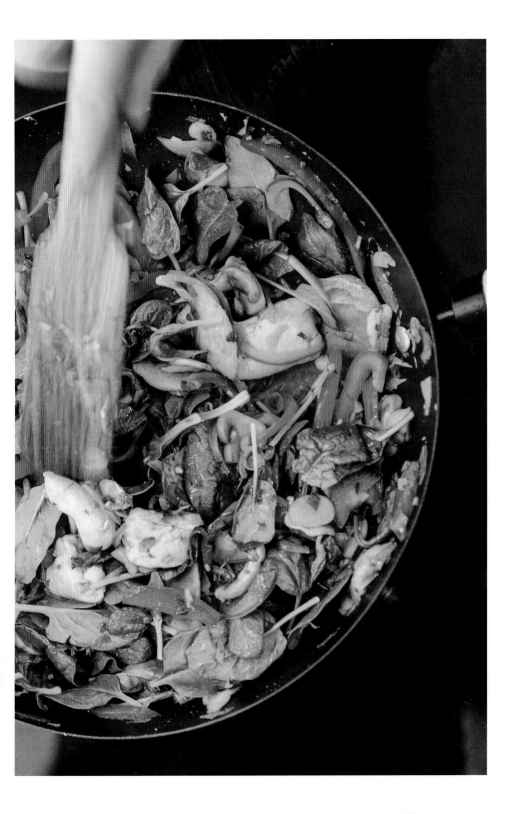

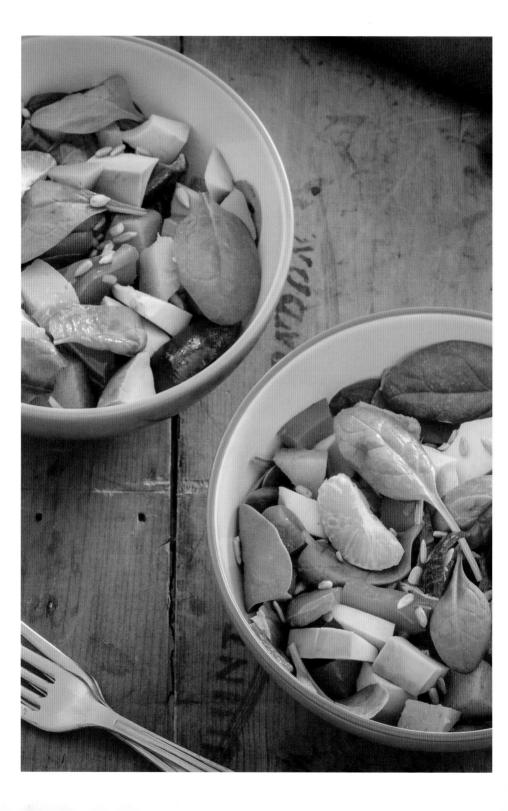

SUPERFOOD SALAD

This salad is especially handy if you get home late at night and don't want to eat a heavy meal. This happens to me all the time. On days when I know it's going to happen, I will have my main meal at lunchtime and then opt for soup or this salad in the evening.

1 Preheat the oven to 180°C/350°F/gas mark 4. Put the butternut squash into a bowl and add in the oil and the ground cumin. Mix everything together with your hands to ensure the squash pieces are evenly coated.

2 Place the squash on a baking tray and put into the preheated oven for 10 minutes.

3 In the meantime, toss the red onion and pepper in the bowl with a drizzle more of oil. Add these to the baking tray with the butternut squash and return to the oven for a further 15 minutes.

4 Prepare the remaining ingredients and place in a large bowl. Remove the roasted squash and vegetables from the oven and add them to the bowl. Toss everything together and serve.

5 This salad will not need a dressing as the mandarin will keep it juicy, as will the butternut squash.

PREP TIME 10 minutes
COOKING TIME 25 minutes
SERVES 2

½ butternut squash, peeled and cut into chunks
1 tbsp rapeseed oil
½ tsp ground cumin
1 red onion, peeled and cut into chunks
1 red pepper, cut into chunks
2 large handfuls of baby spinach or rocket
1 baby avocado, peeled, halved, stoned and chopped into chunks
1 tbsp sunflower seeds, toasted
1 mandarin orange, cut into segments

KARL'S CREAMY CHICKEN AND SWEET POTATO TREAT

This is one of those recipes that tastes like it shouldn't be good for you but actually it is. I have clients who absolutely swear by it for their dinner, and it's surprisingly easy to make. To be honest, it's not glamorous, so don't be surprised if it looks a bit homely – but the taste is knockout!

PREP TIME 5 minutes
COOKING TIME 40 minutes
SERVES 2

2 large sweet potatoes, scrubbed
2 boneless chicken breasts
1 tsp rapeseed oil
1 large onion, peeled and thinly sliced
3 medium leeks, sliced
2 cloves of garlic, peeled and crushed
6 medium mushrooms, sliced
50ml single cream
1 tsp dried oregano
2 handfuls of baby spinach leaves
sea salt and freshly ground black pepper

1 Preheat the oven to 200°C/400°F/gas mark 6.

2 Put the sweet potatoes on a baking tray, pierce the skins with a fork and bake in the oven for 30 minutes. While the potatoes are baking, dice the chicken breasts into roughly 1cm cubes.

3 Heat the rapeseed oil in a large non-stick frying pan and cook the chicken pieces on a high heat until golden brown. When cooked, set aside on a plate lined with a piece of kitchen paper (the kitchen paper will soak up any oil).

4 Put the pan back on a high heat (no need to wash the pan) and add the sliced onion (there should be enough oil left to cook it).

5 When the onion has softened (about 3 minutes), add the sliced leeks, garlic and mushrooms and cook for a further 3 to 5 minutes on a medium heat until everything is soft.

6 Add the cream and oregano. Season to taste and cook for a further 2 minutes on a low heat, stirring gently.

7 Add the cooked chicken and the baby spinach to the mix, cover and bring to a simmer for 2 minutes.

8 Remove the sweet potatoes from the oven after 30 minutes (you can stick a skewer into the middle to test that they're soft right the way through; leave in the oven for a few more minutes if you need to). Dice into 2cm cubes and add to the chicken mix in the pan. Mix through gently and then serve in a deep bowl.

CHILLI CHICKEN PASTA

I love pasta. I love chicken. I love fiery food. This is a combination of all of those loves. It's great for the night before a long run, and when I was doing Ironman Triathlons in my twenties, I ate a LOT of this dish! However, it's also a very tasty and practical dish for a family dinner.

PREP TIME 5 minutes
COOKING TIME 15 minutes
SERVES 2

300g dry brown pasta (penne and fusilli are good shapes for this dish, but you can use whatever you have to hand)
1 tsp rapeseed oil
1 large chicken breast (125 to 150g), cut into 1cm cubes
1 clove of garlic, peeled and crushed
1 medium red pepper, roughly chopped
1 small chilli, deseeded (if you prefer less heat) and finely diced
2 medium tomatoes, roughly chopped
chilli flakes (optional)
sea salt and freshly ground black pepper

1 Cook the pasta according to the packet instructions.

2 While the pasta is cooking, heat the oil in a pan over a high heat. Add the chicken, garlic and red pepper and cook for 1 minute.

3 Reduce the heat to medium and add the chilli to taste (don't add all the chilli if you're nervous about the heat). Season to taste and cook for 6 to 8 minutes until everything has softened down.

4 Add the chopped tomatoes and cook for a further 1 to 2 minutes.

5 By now, the pasta will be cooked or nearly cooked. Check a piece and if it is a little too hard, leave it for another minute or two. (You want it to have a bit of bite left to it – it shouldn't be totally soft, but it shouldn't be chewy either!)

6 Before you drain the pasta, take out a tablespoon of the pasta water and put it to one side. Drain the pasta.

7 Toss together the chicken and veg mix and the pasta and then serve. (Add the reserved pasta water if the chicken and veg mix isn't particularly wet. It will help everything to mix nicely.)

8 Sprinkle a few chilli flakes on top to garnish if you like – you can add as much as you can handle!

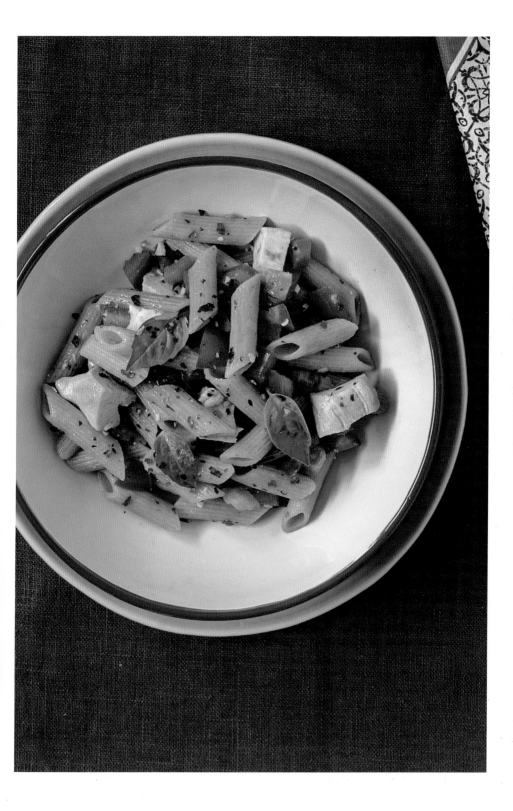

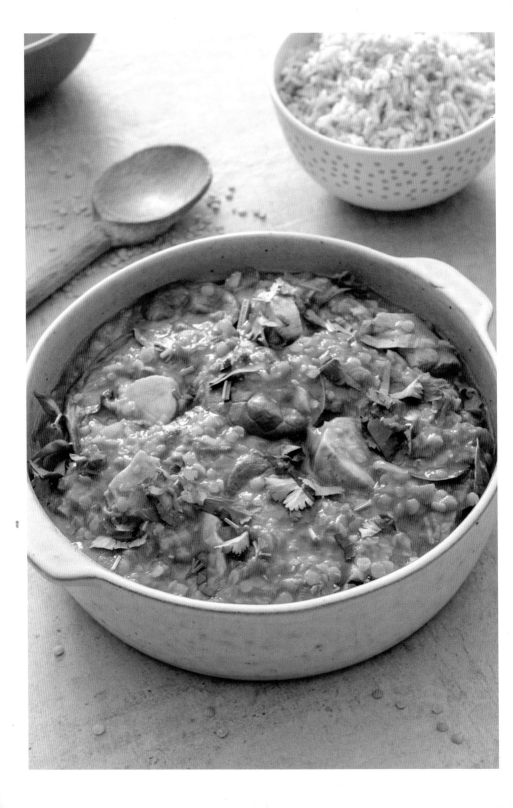

CHICKEN AND RED LENTIL CURRY

Lentils are a fantastic ingredient, yet I used to fear them, as I wasn't sure how to cook them. However, they are an extremely cheap and easy-to-cook ingredient and full of nutrition. So if you've never cooked with lentils before, give this recipe a go and you will see what you have been missing!

1 Put the oil in a large non-stick frying pan or saucepan and heat on high until the oil is hot.

2 Add the onion, garlic and ginger, then reduce the heat to medium and fry until softened. Stir from time to time.

3 Add the chicken, coriander and spices and cook for 5 minutes on a medium heat. Stir occasionally.

4 Add the tomatoes, stock, lentils and coconut milk. Season to taste, stir and then bring to the boil.

5 Reduce the heat to a light simmer and cook for 20 minutes or until the chicken is fully cooked.

6 Lentils really soak up liquid so add a little more water or chicken stock if the sauce is thickening too much and the mix is starting to look heavy or dry.

7 Finally, stir in the spinach, which will wilt down quickly with the heat.

8 Garnish with a few fresh coriander leaves if you like and serve with basmati or brown rice.

PREP TIME 5 minutes
COOKING TIME 30 minutes
SERVES 4

1 tsp rapeseed oil
1 small onion, peeled and finely diced
1 clove of garlic, peeled and crushed
1 knuckle-sized piece of fresh ginger, peeled and finely chopped
4 chicken breasts (125g each!), cut into 2cm pieces
1 tsp chopped coriander, plus extra leaves to garnish (optional)
1 tsp ground cumin
1 tsp ground turmeric
½ tsp chilli powder
1 x 400g tin chopped tomatoes
300ml chicken stock
100g red lentils
200ml low-fat coconut milk
100g baby spinach leaves
sea salt and freshly ground black pepper

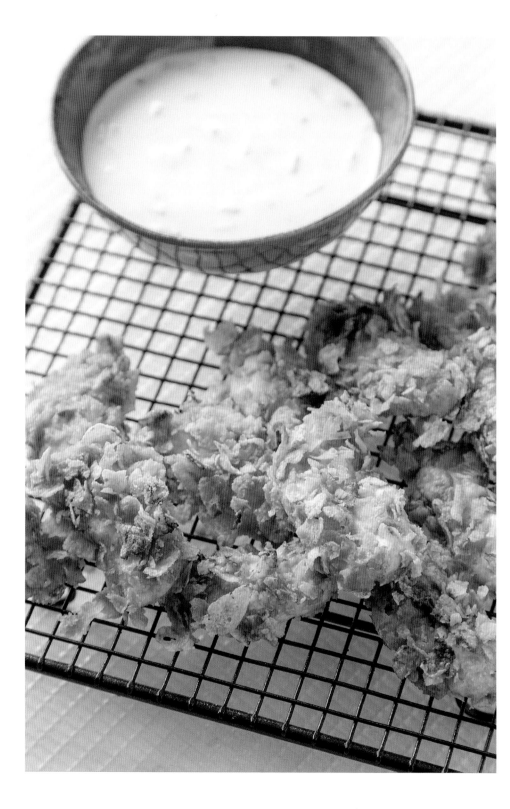

CRISPY CHICKEN GOUJONS

A healthy take on the pub grub classic. I love the goujons from An Súgán in Clonakilty in West Cork, so I thought I'd try to make my own version – perfect for a TV dinner! These are very moreish so are perfect for parties – adults' or children's.

1 Preheat the oven to 180°C/350°F/gas mark 4.

2 Cut the chicken breasts lengthways into thin strips.

3 In a shallow dish, lightly beat the egg, honey and mustard together.

4 Crush the cornflakes in another dish and add a generous grinding of black pepper. Stir the pepper through the cornflake mix.

5 Dip the chicken strips into the egg mixture and then roll in the cornflake mixture to coat.

6 Arrange the chicken strips on a baking tray lined with baking parchment.

7 Put into the preheated oven and bake for 12 minutes. Check one of the goujons. If the chicken is still showing some pink flesh, continue to cook for another few minutes. The chicken flesh should all be white.

8 Mix together all the dip ingredients in a bowl with a fork.

9 Serve the goujons with the lemon and chive dip. You could add a side salad if you're having these as a lunch or light dinner.

PREP TIME 5 minutes
COOKING TIME 15 minutes
SERVES 4

3 large chicken breasts
  (150g each)
1 large egg
1 tbsp honey
1 tsp Dijon or other mild
  mustard
2 to 3 small mugs of
  crushed cornflakes
freshly ground black
  pepper

FOR THE DIP
4 tbsp Greek yoghurt
2 tsp mayonnaise
2 tbsp dried or fresh
  chives
juice of 1 lemon

TURKEY BURGERS

Who doesn't love a good burger? This is my take on the turkey burger craze. They are so flexible that you can make them with anything that's in your fridge.

PREP TIME 5 minutes
COOKING TIME 25 minutes
SERVES 3 to 4

300g lean turkey mince
1 onion, peeled and finely chopped
6 medium mushrooms, finely diced
a few fresh basil leaves, finely chopped
a few fresh coriander leaves, finely chopped
1 tsp Tabasco
1 large egg
sea salt and freshly ground black pepper, to taste
1 tsp rapeseed oil

1 Put all the ingredients into a large bowl and mix together thoroughly using your hands (washed first, of course!).

2 Shape the mix into burgers – you'll make 3 to 4 good-sized burgers from this mix. (If you want to make mini-burgers for children, just make them half the size.)

3 Fry the burgers in a non-stick pan with a little rapeseed oil on a medium heat, or put them under the grill under a medium heat. Cook for 10 to 15 minutes, turning halfway, until cooked through.

4 Serve with a nice mixed salad or even a burger bun with the usual trimmings!

5 These are perfect to freeze, so you could double or triple this recipe and freeze a big batch of uncooked burgers to have your own handy supply of healthy fast food.

LEAN AND JUICY MINCE

This simple yet healthy mince dish is a great way to get some lean protein into your day. It works really well when added to pasta or as a potato or sweet potato topping!

1 Put the oil in a large non-stick frying pan and heat on high until the oil is hot.

2 Add the onion, carrots and red pepper, reduce the heat to medium and cook for 5 minutes, stirring occasionally.

3 Add the garlic and cook for another 5 minutes or so – still stirring from time to time – until the vegetables are soft.

4 Turn the heat back to high, add the mince and cook for 2 minutes, stirring constantly, until the meat is browned.

5 Add the oregano, spices, passata and Tabasco. Season to taste. Bring the mix to the boil, then reduce the heat and simmer gently for 15 minutes.

6 Serve your mince with pasta, rice or a baked potato (regular or sweet) for a delicious, filling, healthy dinner!

PREP TIME 5 minutes
COOKING TIME 30 minutes
SERVES 4

1 tsp rapeseed oil
1 large onion, peeled and finely chopped
2 carrots, peeled and finely chopped
1 red pepper, finely chopped
2 cloves of garlic, peeled and crushed
300g lean mince, either beef or turkey
1 tsp dried oregano
1 tsp grated nutmeg
1 tsp ground cinnamon
1 tsp chilli flakes
300ml passata
a dash of Tabasco – or more if you like it spicy!
sea salt and freshly ground black pepper

BAKED HAKE WITH SWEET POTATO

I know – cooking fish scares you! It used to scare me too. In reality, it isn't scary at all. Once you get your confidence up, you will be cooking fish at least once a week. Try this recipe to get you going.

PREP TIME 5 minutes
COOKING TIME 45 minutes
SERVES 2

1 medium sweet potato, peeled and cut into chunks
2 x 200g hake fillets, skinless
juice of ½ lemon
1 tsp rapeseed oil
200g fresh or frozen green beans
200g fresh or frozen peas
lemon slice and/or chopped parsley to garnish (optional)
sea salt and freshly ground black pepper

1 Preheat the oven to 180°C/350°F/gas mark 4.

2 Put the sweet potato chunks into boiling water, reduce the heat and leave on a strong simmer for about 20 minutes.

3 Line a baking tray with greaseproof paper. Place the hake fillets on the greaseproof paper and season with a little salt and pepper and a squeeze of lemon juice (there's no need to squeeze the lemon in advance, just hold your half lemon in your hand and squeeze the juice out, catching any pips in your other hand; unless your lemon is very small and dry, you can leave a little juice behind to season your final dish).

4 Put the hake onto the middle shelf of the preheated oven and cook for 8 to 10 minutes.

5 While the fish is cooking, heat the rapeseed oil in a wok or ordinary non-stick frying pan on a high heat. When the oil is hot, add the green beans and cook for about 5 minutes so that they're cooked but not soggy. Add the frozen peas for a final 2 minutes' cooking. Season lightly with salt and pepper.

6 Check that the sweet potato is cooked through, then drain it, season to taste and mash it with a fork.

7 Now check your fish. Thicker pieces will take longer to cook, so take the hake out of the oven to check it after 8 minutes (shutting the oven door to retain the heat). If the fish is gently falling apart at the thickest point, it's ready and you can turn off your

oven. If not, put it back into the oven for another minute or two.

8 Divide the mash between two plates. Place the hake fillets partly resting on the mash and serve your green veg alongside (you can be fancier if serving friends by putting the mash in the centre with the fish on top and scattering the green veg all around). Add a final light squeeze of lemon juice over everything.

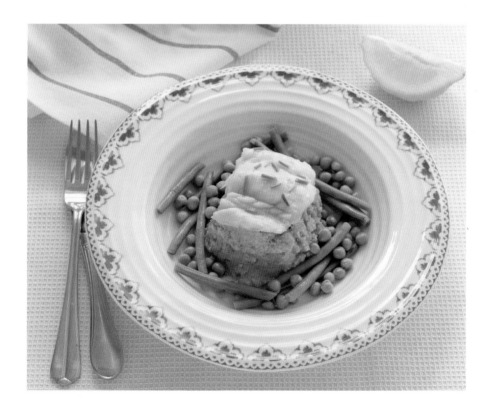

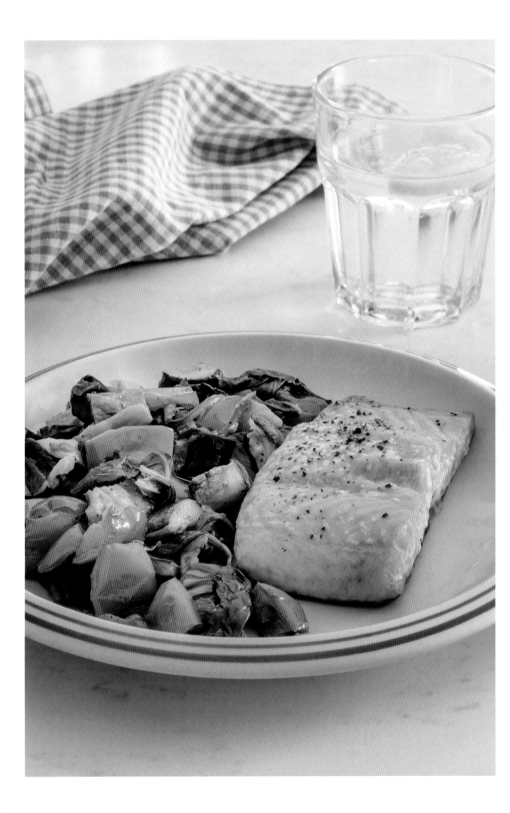

BAKED SALMON WITH MEDITERRANEAN VEGETABLES

Salmon is a great source of protein and healthy fats and is great for your body – but I have to admit that I don't eat it! This is a recipe that my wife makes and it always smells delicious. With so many people eating salmon, I wanted to share it in the book.

1 Preheat the oven to 200°C/400°F/gas mark 6.

2 Place the chopped aubergine, courgette, red pepper and red onion in a bowl, then add the rosemary and olive oil, season and mix it all together with your hands.

3 Spread out the coated vegetables on a baking tray lined with baking parchment and put into the preheated oven for about 8 minutes.

4 Now push the vegetables to one side and put the salmon fillets in the middle of the baking tray, season with pepper and return to the oven for a further 10 minutes.

5 Check that the salmon fillets are cooked through – the colour will be pale pink all over and if you poke them with a knife, the flesh will be coming apart slightly – and then remove from the oven. Mix the spinach through the cooked veg – the leaves will wilt down in the heat – and serve.

6 This is a simple lunch or after-work dinner that takes very little time and is really satisfying and packed full of nutrition. I only wish I could get on board with salmon so I could eat it myself!

PREP TIME 10 minutes
COOKING TIME 20 minutes
SERVES 2

½ aubergine, chopped
  into 2cm chunks
1 small courgette,
  chopped into 2cm
  chunks
1 red pepper, chopped
  into 2cm chunks
1 red onion, peeled and
  chopped into 2cm
  chunks
1 tsp dried rosemary
1 tbsp olive oil
2 salmon fillets (approx
  150g each)
2 handfuls of baby
  spinach leaves
sea salt and freshly
  ground black pepper

HEALTHY ROAST VEGETABLE LASAGNE

Whenever we have a group of friends coming over, the large dish comes out and I am into lasagne mode – healthy, hearty and full of goodness!

PREPTIME 10 minutes
COOKING TIME 1 hour
SERVES 4

1 medium red pepper, roughly chopped
1 medium yellow pepper, roughly chopped
1 medium green pepper, roughly chopped
1 medium carrot, unpeeled but washed, chopped into 2cm chunks
1 medium courgette, chopped into 2cm chunks
1 pack of mushrooms, roughly sliced
2 tbsp rapeseed oil
1 x 200g pack of cherry tomatoes, halved
300ml passata
1 x 50g pack washed baby leaf spinach
300ml Greek yoghurt
250g ricotta cheese
freshly grated nutmeg (optional)
1 x 500g pack wholegrain lasagne sheets

1 Preheat the oven to 180°C/350°F/gas mark 4.

2 Line a large roasting tray with baking parchment and put in the chopped peppers, carrot, courgette and mushrooms (it doesn't matter how big or small the vegetables are chopped as long as they are all about the same size so they roast evenly).

3 Drizzle the oil over the vegetables and stir so they are all evenly coated. Spread out the veg into an even layer and put the roasting tray into the preheated oven for about 20 minutes until the veg are roasted (you can check after 15 to make sure they're not drying out).

4 Drain off any excess liquid that might have come from the mushrooms cooking down and then add the halved cherry tomatoes for the final 5 minutes of cooking time.

5 Once you remove the roasted veg from the oven, pour the passata over them, scatter the spinach leaves on top, season lightly and stir. (Leave the oven on while you do this, as you'll be using it again shortly.)

6 Mix the yoghurt and ricotta together in a small bowl and season with a little salt, pepper and the nutmeg, if using. (Just add a little nutmeg at first to see if it's to your taste – about half a teaspoon. You can always add more next time you cook the recipe until you find the right amount for you!)

7 To assemble, spread even layers of each of the elements in a lasagne dish in this order: yoghurt/ricotta; lasagne sheets; roasted veg; yoghurt/ricotta; lasagne sheets; roasted veg; yoghurt/ricotta; lasagne sheets.

8 Top with the finely grated Cheddar or Parmesan.

9 Pop in the oven for 40 to 45 minutes until the lasagne sheets are cooked and the sauces are bubbling.

10 Serve with a nice simple salad to really ramp up your intake of healthy veg.

TOPPING

50g extra-mature Cheddar or Parmesan, finely grated

sea salt and freshly ground black pepper

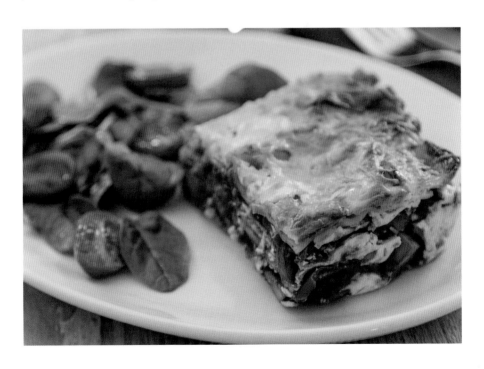

A HEARTY HOTPOT

I can't really call this one a fast food, but it's so delicious and so healthy that I couldn't leave it out! It's a great take on a classic beef and red wine stew. I make a large pot of it, divide it into portions and then freeze them. If you follow my example, you'll always have this stew when you feel the need for something comforting!

PREP TIME 15 minutes
COOKING TIME 2 hours
SERVES 8

2 tbsp rapeseed oil
1 large onion, peeled and roughly chopped
3 cloves of garlic, peeled and finely chopped
300g mushrooms, roughly chopped
1.5kg round steak, chopped into 2cm cubes
250ml red wine
250ml chicken stock
2 tbsp red wine vinegar
4 large sweet potatoes, peeled and chopped into 2cm chunks
sea salt and freshly ground black pepper

1 Preheat the oven to 160°C/325°F/gas mark 3.

2 Heat the oil over a medium heat in a large ovenproof casserole or saucepan.

3 Add the onions and cook gently until soft, generally 8 to 10 minutes. Now add the garlic and mushrooms and cook for another minute or so.

4 Add the steak and brown it completely – this should take about 2 minutes – before adding the wine, chicken stock and vinegar and seasoning to taste.

5 Stir, then increase the heat and bring the mixture to the boil.

6 Remove from the heat, cover the pot or saucepan with a lid and put into the centre of the oven.

7 After 1 hour, put the sweet potatoes in a pot of boiling water. Cook on a medium heat, at a simmer, until they are tender – about 15 to 20 minutes. When cooked, remove from the heat, drain, add a little salt and pepper to taste and mash with a fork or potato masher.

8 After 90 minutes of cooking, remove the casserole dish from the oven. Increase the oven temperature to 200°C/400°F/gas mark 6.

9 Uncover the dish. (Remember, everything will be very hot so be careful to use good oven gloves and

take care to avoid the hot steam when removing the lid.) Spoon the sweet potato mash over the stew in a thick layer and press the surface with a fork to make ridges on the top.

10 Place the casserole dish back in the oven for 20 minutes, until the mash is crisp and beginning to brown. Serve on its own or with a fresh, healthy salad on the side.

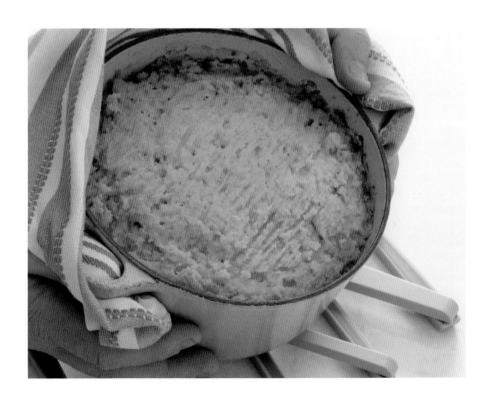

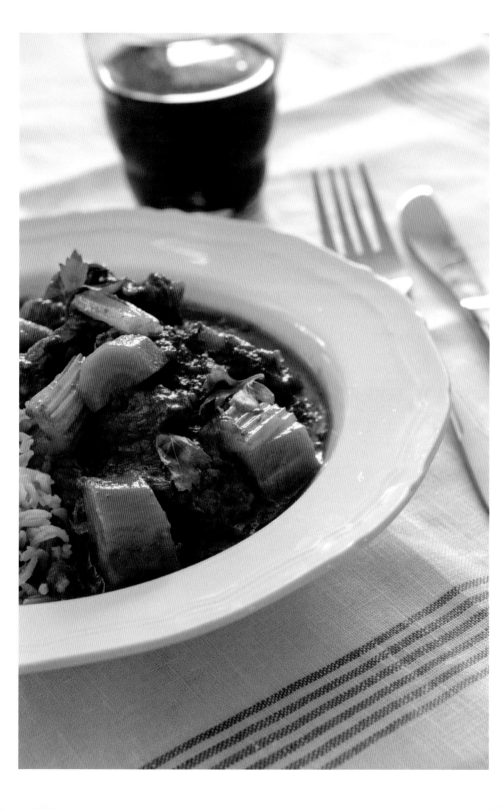

BEEF AND GUINNESS STEW

Again, not a quick one, but it's an absolute classic. What's great about it is that it's very quick to throw together and it tastes like you've been slaving over it for hours, so it's perfect if you have guests! It's another one that freezes very well.

1 Preheat the oven to 160°C/325°F/gas mark 3.

2 Heat the oil over a medium heat in a large ovenproof casserole or saucepan.

3 Add the chopped onion and cook gently until soft, generally 8 to 10 minutes. Now add the garlic, carrots, celery and mushrooms and cook for another minute or so.

4 Add the steak and brown it completely – it should take about 2 minutes – before adding the Guinness, tomatoes and chicken stock and seasoning to taste.

5 Stir, then increase the heat and bring the mixture to the boil.

6 Remove from the heat, cover the pot or saucepan with a lid and put into the centre of the oven.

7 Leave it for 2 hours (walk the dog… go for a run!).

8 When you return, you'll end up with a wonderfully rich, comforting stew.

9 Serve with potatoes, sweet potatoes or brown rice.

PREP TIME 15 minutes
COOKING TIME 2 hours 20 minutes
SERVES 8

2 tbsp rapeseed oil
1 large onion, peeled and finely chopped
3 cloves of garlic, peeled and finely chopped
6 large carrots, peeled and finely chopped
4 sticks of celery, finely chopped
300g mushrooms, finely chopped
1.5kg round steak, chopped into 2cm cubes
250ml Guinness
1 x 400g tin chopped tomatoes
250ml chicken stock
sea salt and freshly ground black pepper

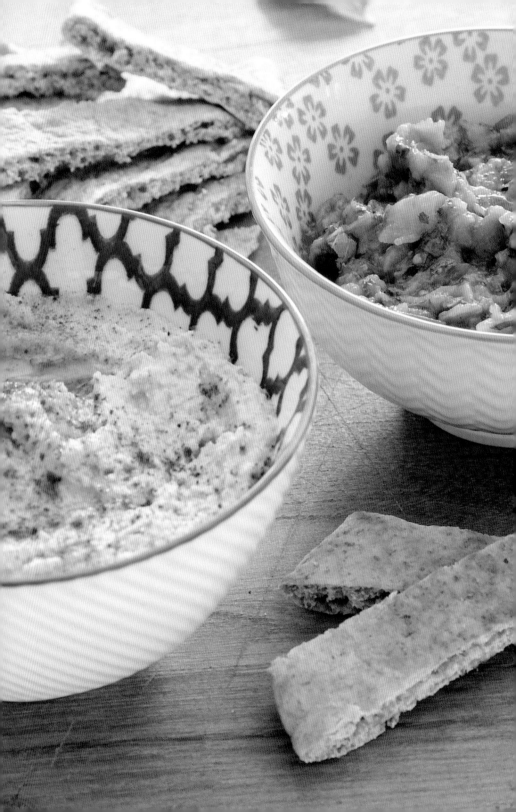

SNACKS AND TREATS

14

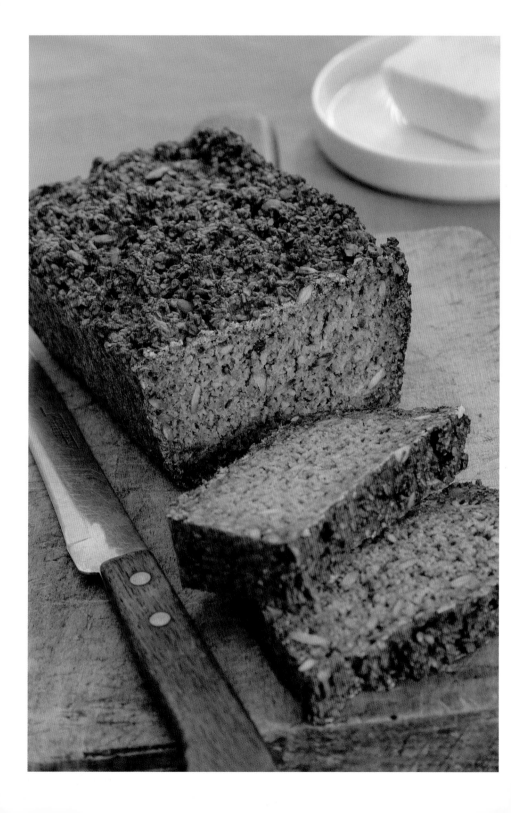

JEAN'S BROWN BREAD

This is my wife's yummy brown bread recipe, which is so much nicer and better than any you will buy in the supermarket. Full of seeds and oats, it's a winner!

1 Preheat the oven to 180°C/350°F/gas mark 4.

2 Prepare a 900g loaf tin by greasing the insides thoroughly with butter or lining it with greaseproof paper.

3 Stir the yoghurt, beaten egg and treacle together in a mixing bowl.

4 Now add the oats, seeds and bread soda (make sure you rub it through your hands to eliminate any lumps, or use a small sieve). Stir these thoroughly through the yoghurt mix.

5 Pour the mix into the prepared loaf tin and level the top with a knife, sprinkle with oats and put into the centre of the oven to bake for 30 minutes.

6 After 30 minutes, reduce the oven temperature to 150°C/300°F/gas mark 2 and bake for a further 30 minutes.

7 If you tap the base when you take the loaf out of the tin you should get a nice hollow sound. Leave the loaf to cool on a wire rack.

8 This bread is perfect with soups, salads and dips.

PREP TIME 10 minutes
COOKING TIME 1 hour
MAKES 1 x 900g loaf

500ml natural yoghurt
1 large egg, beaten
1 tbsp treacle
300g jumbo porridge
oats, plus extra for
sprinkling
4 tbsp mixed seeds
(e.g. sunflower,
pumpkin, poppy)
2 tsp bread soda

QUICK AND SIMPLE HUMMUS

Hummus is not just a delicious party dip, it's also great as a healthy snack with some sliced vegetables during the day. This traditional Middle Eastern dip is usually made from chickpeas, tahini (crushed sesame seed paste) and olive oil but apart from an optional drizzle on top, my version omits the olive oil and you also avoid the excessive salt that's added to the shop-bought versions. This simple recipe is a winner on both taste and health!

PREP TIME 5 minutes
SERVES 2 as a dip

1 x 400g tin chickpeas, drained and rinsed (reserve the liquid from the tin)
1 tbsp tahini paste or unsweetened peanut butter
1 clove of garlic, peeled and crushed
juice of ½ large lemon
½ tsp ground cumin
50ml cold water

1 Blitz everything together in a food processor. (If you don't have a food processor, you can use a liquidizer – add the chickpeas and tahini first, then everything else. Or, of course, you can simply mash everything together with a fork. It's a lot more elbow grease and the end result will be rougher, but it's how it was made in olden times.)

2 Add a little of the reserved chickpea liquid if the mixture is too dry and continue to add liquid (either the chickpea liquid or just water) tablespoon by tablespoon until you get a consistency you're happy with.

3 To serve, drizzle a little extra virgin olive oil over the top and sprinkle with some smoked paprika if you have it.

4 This hummus will go beautifully with the Prawn Kebabs (see recipe on page xx) or as a spread with Jean's Brown Bread (page xx). But, frankly, the only limit to using hummus is your imagination.

(See image on page 128)

BABA GANOUSH

I love Middle Eastern food and it can be so easy to make too. Baba ganoush is a traditional dip that's based on roasted aubergines. It usually includes tahini but my version omits that, so you end up with a very light and delicate mash – another delicious addition to both your party-food and healthy-snack options!

1 Preheat the oven to 200°C/400°F/gas mark 6.

2 Line a baking tray (or roasting tin) with baking parchment.

3 Prick the skins of the aubergines with a fork. Place them on the baking tray and put into the middle of the oven to roast for approximately 25 to 30 minutes.

4 While the aubergines are roasting, heat 1 tablespoon of the olive oil in a frying pan over a low heat. Gently fry the cherry tomatoes for about 10 minutes or until they have started to break down and are lovely and soft.

5 After 25 to 30 minutes, the aubergines should be soft and collapsing. Take them out of the oven and allow to cool slightly.

6 Scoop out the aubergine flesh and discard the skins. Sieve the flesh over a bowl to allow any juices to drain off and then finely chop the drained flesh.

7 Mix together the chopped aubergine flesh, tomatoes, mint, lemon juice and the remaining 3 tablespoons of the olive oil. Check the taste and add seasoning if needed. Serve with some raw vegetable crudités, brown pitta or on some of Jean's lovely brown bread (see page 131).

(See image on page 128)

PREP TIME 10 minutes
COOKING TIME 45 minutes
SERVES 4 as a dip

2 large aubergines, whole
4 tbsp extra virgin olive oil
200g cherry tomatoes, quartered
15g fresh mint, finely chopped
juice of 1 lemon
sea salt and freshly ground black pepper

FLAPJACKS

These are a great snack when out for a hill walk or a cycle, or as a snack during the day.

PREP TIME 5 minutes
COOKING TIME 20 minutes
MAKES 12 flapjacks

100g jumbo porridge oats
100g nuts of your choice,
  roughly chopped
1 tbsp flaxseeds
  (or linseeds)
75g dates, roughly
  chopped (Medjool dates
  are nice if you can get
  them)
50g dried apricots,
  roughly chopped
1 tbsp rapeseed oil
100g honey

1 Preheat the oven to 160°C/325°F/gas mark 3.

2 Line a 20cm square baking tray with baking parchment.

3 Mix all the dry ingredients together in a large bowl. Then add the oil and honey and mix thoroughly.

4 Transfer the mixture to the baking tray, spread evenly and flatten firmly using the back of a spoon.

5 Put into the preheated oven and bake for 20 minutes.

6 Remove from the oven and mark out 12 rectangles before they cool down.

7 Allow to cool completely, then turn out of the tray and break into 12 individual flapjacks. Store in an airtight container in a cool place. They will keep for up to 10 days.

(Flapjacks are at the front in the picture.)

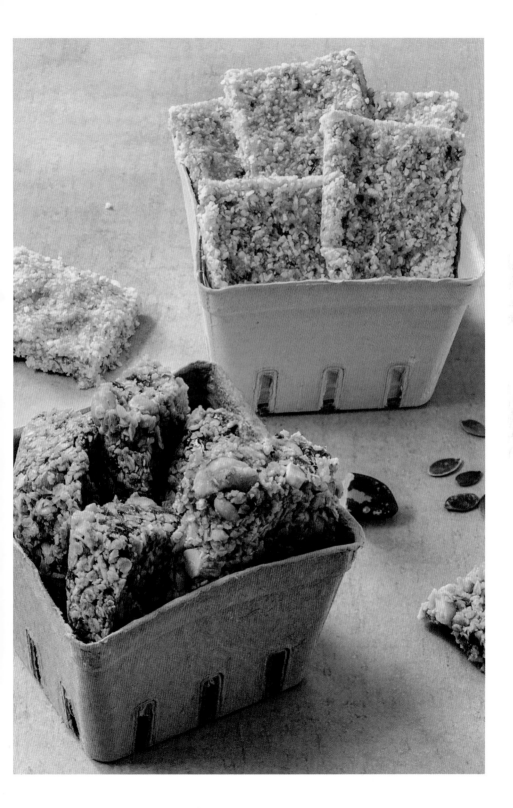

FRUIT 'N' NUT SQUARES

Here is another great, healthy snack that is simple to make – you don't even have to bake it – and it lasts in the fridge for over a week. The flavour will remind you of a Bounty or Macaroon bar, and it is a good option for a lunchbox (a child's or grown-up's!) instead of sweets or crisps.

PREP TIME 5 minutes
MAKES 12 squares

100g almonds (whole, blanched or flaked – whatever you can get)
65g cashew nuts
100g desiccated coconut
12 dates, pitted
1 to 2 tbsp coconut oil

1 Line a 20cm square or rectangular baking tin with baking parchment.

2 Blitz the almonds, cashew nuts and coconut together in a food processor until everything is small and fine but not powdery (about 20 seconds).

3 Add the dates and blitz for another 20 to 30 seconds.

4 Finally, add the coconut oil and blitz until the mixture just comes together. Don't over-blend or the oils in the nuts will start to separate out and the texture will be wrong (think nut butter!).

5 Transfer the mixture into the prepared tin and refrigerate for 30 minutes, then remove and cut into 12 squares. (If you are making this with children's lunchboxes in mind you could divide the mixture into even smaller pieces – say, 16 – for smaller tummies.)

6 Your fruit 'n' nut treats will keep in a sealed container in the fridge for up to 10 days.

(Fruit'n'Nut Squares are pictured at the back of the picture on the previous page.)

CHOCOLATEY NUTS

This may sound naughty, but it's a very healthy treat – full of protein and selenium from the Brazil nuts and antioxidants from the dark chocolate. Just remember that it's a snack, so enjoy in moderation!

1 Line a baking tray or large plate with baking parchment.

PREP TIME 15 minutes
MAKES 250g

2 Break the chocolate into pieces and put it into a bowl. Put the bowl over a saucepan of gently simmering water. The bowl should be bigger than the saucepan rim so that it sits in the saucepan, but the bottom of the bowl remains above the level of the water, rather than touching it.

200g Brazil nuts
50g good-quality dark
    chocolate (70% cocoa
    solids)

3 Allow the chocolate to melt gently, stirring occasionally – it should take around 3 minutes. (Ensure you don't get any water into the chocolate, as water will damage its smooth consistency.)

4 Once the chocolate has melted, dip each Brazil nut into it so that one end is thoroughly coated.

5 Transfer the chocolate-coated nuts to the baking parchment and allow to set.

6 Store in a sealed container in a cool place and your chocolatey nuts will keep for up to seven days.

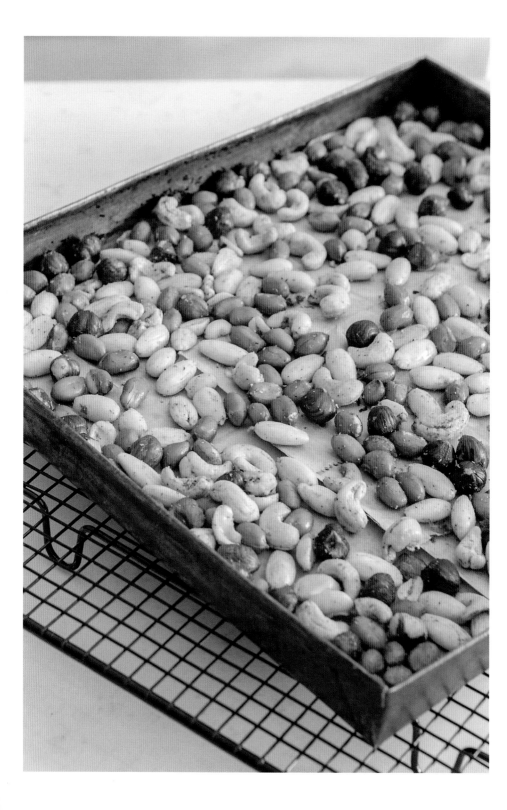

TANDOORI MIXED NUTS

Nuts are full of protein and minerals and are super-handy as a snack. Remember, snack size is about a handful (assuming you don't have huge hands and that you fill your hand loosely!).

1 Preheat the oven to 180°C/350°F/gas mark 4.

2 Line a baking tray with baking parchment.

3 Mix the nuts, the oil and the garam masala together in a bowl.

4 Transfer the mixture to the baking tray and spread out evenly. Put the tray into the preheated oven and roast for 8 to 10 minutes.

5 Remove from the oven and allow to cool. Store in a sealed container and your Tandoori mixed nuts will last for up to 10 days.

6 They're delicious as a snack with a drink watching TV – just remember to put out a small bowl for yourself rather than the whole lot!

PREP TIME 5 minutes
COOKING TIME 10 minutes
MAKES 400g

100g unsalted peanuts
100g unsalted cashews
100g unsalted almonds
100g unroasted hazelnuts
1 tsp rapeseed oil
2 tsp garam masala

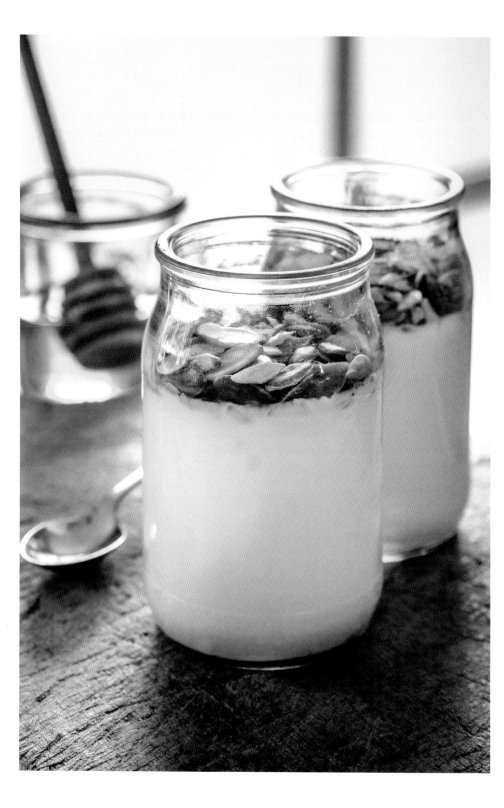

YOGHURT AND SEED POTS

These pots are great in the morning when you're rushing out the door, to grab and go and bring into work. I also use them as snacks for large groups – they're super-quick to make and healthy too!

1 Drizzle the honey over the yoghurt and sprinkle with the seeds.

PREP TIME 2 minutes
SERVES 1

2 For a more interesting flavour, dry-roast half the seeds in a pan (i.e. heat the pan without any oil and toast the seeds for a minute or two, making sure not to burn them). That way you get a nice toasty flavour while retaining the nutritional benefits of the raw seeds.

2 tsp honey
125g Greek yoghurt
25g mixed seeds (e.g. pumpkin, sesame, sunflower)

3 When we were photographing this recipe, we happened to have some flaked almonds available, so we added them. They made a nice addition.

4 If this is a snack you like to have regularly, you could batch-roast some seeds for quicker preparation.

FROZEN YOGHURT

A great alternative to ice cream and one that is great fun to make too. Get your yoghurt, choose your fruit and off you go!

PREP TIME 5 minutes
SERVES 4

280g frozen raspberries
(or any other berries
of your choice – or a
mixture!)
2 tbsp honey
100g Greek yoghurt

1 Put all the ingredients into a food processor or blender and blitz for 60 to 90 seconds. Check to ensure there aren't any lumpy bits, and if there are, just stir the mixture and blend for another 30 seconds.

2 Pour the mixture into an airtight container and then put it straight into the freezer for at least 3 hours. It's that easy!

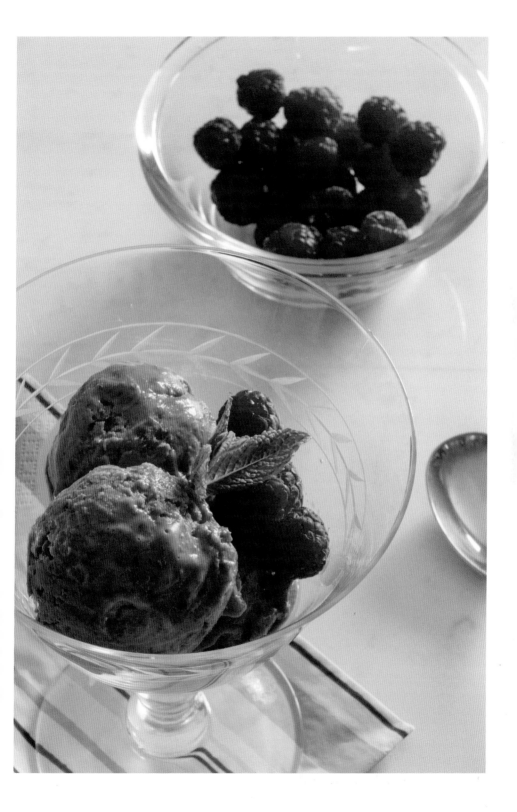

APPLE CRUMBLE

While I'm not really into desserts, I am partial to an apple crumble. The most amazing I have ever tasted came from the kitchen of Mary Flahavan of the legendary Flahavan family. So this is inspired by Mary's recipe, which she very kindly gave me permission to use. It's the pièce de résistance to finish the recipe section of the book!

PREP TIME 15 minutes
COOKING TIME 40 minutes
SERVES 6 people

FOR THE FILLING
675g apples, peeled, cored and chopped into 1cm chunks
75g caster sugar

FOR THE CRUMBLE
75g plain flour
75g jumbo porridge oats
75g light brown sugar
75g butter

1 Preheat the oven to 180°C/350°F/gas mark 4.

2 First, prepare the filling. Put the chopped apples into a large baking dish and sprinkle with the sugar.

3 To make the crumble topping, combine the flour, oats, sugar and butter in a food processor until they resemble coarse breadcrumbs. Do this carefully so you get a crumbly rather than a powdery texture – pulse the food processor rather than turning it on full. (You can do this by hand if you don't have a food processor. Just rub the butter into the flour and sugar with your thumbs and forefingers until it's crumbly and then mix in the oats.)

4 Now sprinkle the crumble mixture over the apples and bake in the preheated oven for 40 minutes until the crumble is crisp and browning on top and the filling is bubbling round the edges.

5 Delicious with some creamy Greek yoghurt!

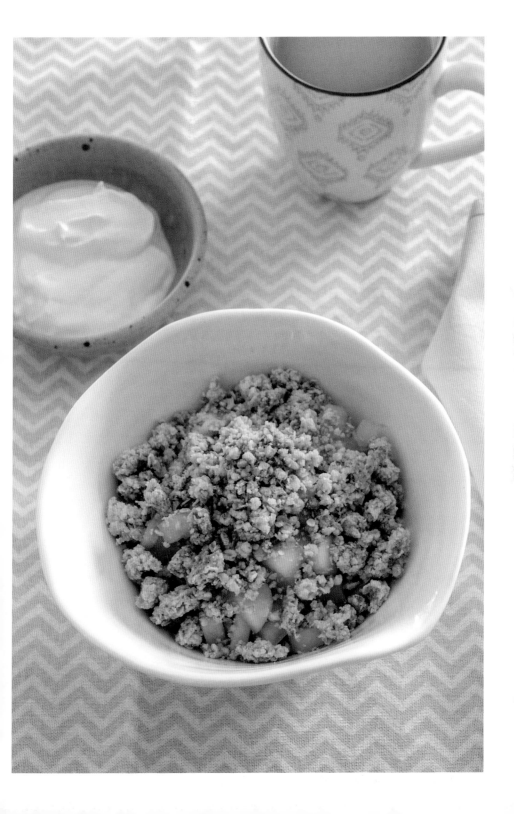

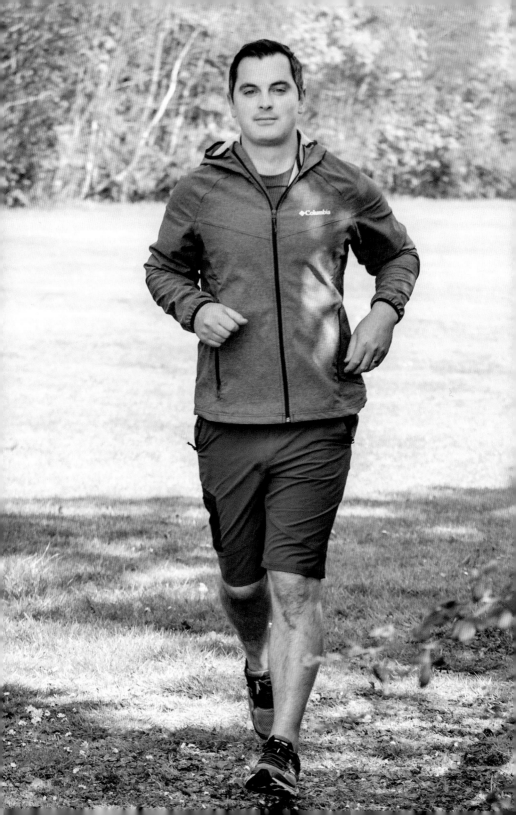

Fitness

The body is an amazing machine that needs to be used, challenged and maintained.

15 WHAT'S YOUR BODY TYPE?

Before I get into the nitty-gritty of exercise, this would be a good moment for you to identify your body type. By figuring that out, you will understand a lot more about how you respond to exercise and diet and where you store your weight. Understanding your body type may help you to make sense of certain patterns – for instance, why you and your best friend eat more or less the same way and do the same amount of activity, but they never put on any weight and you put it on very easily. (Life isn't fair sometimes and you're just going to have to get over it! And as you'll see below, naturally thin people aren't necessarily healthier than those who have to be more careful about their weight.)

Identifying your body type will help you to make your exercise more specific and ensure that you get the most out of workouts. (I mention different types of exercise such as resistance work, cardio training and interval training below. I will go into detail about these in the chapters that follow. 'Reps' means the number of repetitions of a movement in an exercise.)

Remember that no matter what body type you are, with exercise and healthy eating, you will begin to change your life.

MALE BODY TYPES

I describe three male body shapes here, but of course many, if not most, people are a mixture of two (for instance, I am a mixture of mesomorph and endomorph).

Endomorph: Visually the physique is quite rounded and smooth, with very little definition. You are prone to gaining weight quickly and easily. One of the reasons for this is that you may have a slow metabolism and the number of calories you burn on a daily basis is naturally on the low side.

Simple changes in what you eat will make a big impact on how you feel, your digestion and your weight. Equally, you will find that it is easy to gain bulk with training.

This is a great physique for strength and power, but it can be extremely frustrating when trying to lose weight. For you, focusing on food is 80 per cent of your results. While it's always the case that you can't out-train a bad diet, it is especially the case if you have this body type.

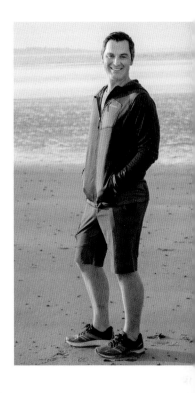

Moderate heart-rate endurance exercise – exercise that gets your heart rate to around 70 per cent of its maximum (where you are out of breath but still able to chat) – is fantastic for this body type, along with resistance work with a medium repetitions range of 12, 15 or 20 reps.

Ectomorph: Ectomorphs have very fast metabolic rates, are generally very slim, despite eating whatever they want, and struggle to put on weight. This may seem ideal, but the truth is that ectomorphs tend to eat worse foods than most, and can have high levels of dangerous visceral fat around the midriff and other diet-related issues. For ectomorphs it can be incredibly hard to gain weight and to gain lean muscle tissue.

Remember that no matter what body type you are, with exercise and healthy eating, you will begin to change your life.

The way forward is to eat meals every two to three hours and to eat protein with every meal. This, combined with an exercise plan with a lower repetitions range will increase your lean muscle tissue, reduce your fat levels and help you get healthier, though it will take some time so you need to be patient.

Mesomorph: This is a mixture of the two other body types. It can be easy to get stronger, get results and lose weight. The mesomorph metabolism is generally high and, when your food is good, the weight will decrease quite quickly. But you can gain weight quickly too, so you need to keep the food right.

Most people will fall into this category, shaping up relatively quickly and seeing improvements in tone and weight quite fast too.

FEMALE BODY TYPES

Women can be one of the three body types above, but as there are more variations for women, this list is more tailored to female bodies. Just like men, you can often be a mixture of the different types, but take a look through these four below and see which one seems right for your body.

Celery: Your hips and shoulders are the same width, you have a slim body and a fast metabolism, meaning that you can almost eat whatever you like and your weight is pretty much stable all year round. While this sounds great, it can be frustrating if you would prefer a curvier shape. Also, because you can eat whatever you want, your diet can be unhealthy – you may be slim but you will lack tone and have plenty of visceral fat.

To get a curvier shape, you need to hit the gym and do resistance exercises such as press-ups, squats and lunges, or pretty much anything with low–medium repetition range. It will increase your lean muscle tissue. Eating regularly to try to offset the speed of your metabolism – every two to three hours – is important too.

Apple: This is a typical Irish and British body shape and probably the most dangerous type too. Before I explain why, let me tell you the good news: you will get fast results from changing your lifestyle.

If you're an apple, you store most of your weight around the middle of your body from your chest to your pelvis, and often have slim legs and arms. The apple shape can increase with age as your metabolism slows down and your body develops fat around the mid-section. This is especially dangerous because you tend to have a high level of visceral fat, lots of stomach bloating and poor digestion.

Getting healthy is incredibly important for you and once you start, you will see numbers changing quickly. If this body type describes you, then aim to do plenty of cardio training and fast, light weights with high repetitions, and follow the food recommendations. Hard work will yield great results and for you, your waist measurement is an especially important indicator of health, so don't avoid that tape measure, whatever you do!

Pear: Pear is a typical Latin physique but also one that we are seeing more in Ireland. You can gain weight quite fast, your hips are wider than your shoulders and you have gained weight on your hips over the years. You find it hard to lose fat and if you've tried weights before, you found that your jeans didn't get any looser.

Workouts with heavy weights won't help, so you need to mix it up with interval training, using alternating speeds of cardiovascular training, combined with light-weight workouts featuring exercises such as side leg raises, bum kicks and pelvic floor kicks. These are great for you, obviously combined with a good diet.

Apple - This is a typical Irish and British body shape and probably the most dangerous type too ... but let me tell you the good news: you will get fast results from changing your lifestyle.

Sometimes you will find that you suffer from fluid retention too. If this is the case, then you need to increase your effort levels in your exercise sessions and drink more water during the day. Lemons, limes or apple cider vinegar are all great when added to your water, as they all naturally help to counter fluid retention.

Hourglass: Because of its even proportions and defined shape, this body type – with broad shoulders, a narrow waist and hips that are a similar width to the shoulders – has always been fashionable on the silver screen and in fashion, and it's one that many of my female clients want when they come in for their first meeting.

If you're a natural hourglass body type, your weight can go up or down quite quickly depending on your diet, as your body is incredibly sensitive to the foods that you eat, and when you knuckle down, you can get into good shape very easily. Your metabolism is consistent and when you improve your diet, your weight/shape also improves very quickly.

The best exercises are boot-camp-style hard workouts combined with cardiovascular sessions, helping to get your waist back into shape and get your lean tissue levels up. Repetitions across all ranges will work well here; I normally use 15 to 20 reps with my clients and find that these get the best results.

FIT PEOPLE STAY YOUNGER & LIVE LONGER!

16

We know that people who exercise and move more on a regular basis live longer, have reduced risk of cardiovascular disease and metabolic disorders and are happier than those who don't. This is not a coincidence; the body is an amazing machine that needs to be used, challenged and maintained. Just like a car needs to be driven regularly to work at its best, our bodies need this too. Our ancestors thousands of years ago walked, ran, jumped, crouched, stretched, lifted and carried. We couldn't be further from that.

In order to get more energy into your day, you have to move more and push your body. If you feel tired all the time, then take a look at your activity levels. Chances are they are very low. You need to move more and move hard enough to get slightly out of breath to get the maximum benefits. The hormonal release when you exercise will not only give you more energy so you will feel better and work better during the day, but you will sleep better at night too.

Exercise is basically any movement at all. Once you are moving and getting your heart rate up, then you are exercising. Any exercise in your day is an improvement, no matter what it is and no matter how much or how little you have done.

If you can combine this movement with measurement – like those I gave you in Chapter 2, page 20: resting heart rate, waist measurement, weight – you will begin to see exactly what is happening as a result of your training. As I said already, measurement is probably the single best way of motivating yourself. It proves that what you are doing is actually having an effect, and we all love to see the numbers move and the progress we're making.

- The lower your resting heart rate, the better your aerobic fitness will be and the healthier you will be.

- If you can begin to get your waist measurement down, lowering the amount of fat stored around your midriff, the more you will reduce your risk of cardiovascular disease and the healthier you will be.

To the scales, 1lb of fat tissue is the same as 1lb of muscle tissue. But in our bodies, fat and muscle are very different.

- As for weight, when it comes to measuring fat and muscle, the weighing scales are neutral. To the scales, 1lb of fat tissue is the same as 1lb of muscle tissue. But in our bodies, fat and muscle are very different. Fat is spread out and soft and takes up a lot of space. Muscle tissue, on the other hand, is tightly packed and firm and takes up less space. That's why two people can have the same number on the scales but their bodies can look quite different. Unfortunately, exercising alone won't get rid of excess fat. But if you are overweight and start improving your diet, the number coming down on the scales will be a sign that you are reducing your fat stores, and if you combine this with exercise, you will also be improving your ratio of fat to muscle and, again, the healthier you will be.

Exercise helps you to maintain your weight by making your body more efficient at burning energy. That's because muscle is high-maintenance tissue that burns fuel at a high rate. So muscle uses up more of the calories you provide when you eat. And if you exercise consistently and keep your muscles maintained, you help to increase the rate at which your body is using up calories – your metabolism. This is particularly important as you get older.

Many people feel that getting older is an excuse to sit more and move less. The reality is that as you age, you need to keep moving. By increasing the amount of exercise you do, the type of exercise you do and eating more healthily, you can help to future-proof your health.

Here are just some of the things that will happen as you age (and I'm not talking about becoming a pensioner – this is a process that commences in your thirties!):

- Your metabolism slows down.
- You gain fat mass.
- You lose muscle mass.
- Your bone density decreases and you are at increased risk of osteoporosis (thinning bones), leading to fractures later in life.
- You are at an increased risk of arthritis.

Not only does maintaining your muscle mass help in managing your weight, it is also crucial for general and bone health as you get older. The same weight-bearing exercise we do to maintain muscle is also needed to maintain bone. But the more you maintain your muscle mass, the stronger and more energetic you will feel, and the greater your capacity to do the kind of weight-bearing exercise that is necessary to stay healthy. As you can see, it's all a virtuous cycle!

There really is no reason not to improve your physical and mental health, and to combat the effects of ageing, by using the tools in this book, no matter what age you are. The next chapter will outline the three different types of fitness you need to think about.

Many people feel that getting older is an excuse to sit more and move less. The reality is that as you age, you need to keep moving.

17 THE THREE-PRONGED APPROACH TO GETTING FIT

The good news – or maybe the bad news, depending on your personality – is that just like with diet, there is no one-shot simple way of becoming fitter. You'll have to give it a little thought and attention. To repeat the image I've used a few times already, our bodies are sophisticated machines, so keeping ourselves well tuned requires a few different strategies. However, this does not mean that getting or staying fit is complicated or difficult. Put simply, fitness rests on three legs – resistance or strength training, cardiovascular or aerobic training and passive training. Take away one aspect and your programme will be a bit unbalanced. Once you understand the role of each aspect, you can mix and match elements across the week to fit in with your lifestyle and schedule and to keep things varied and interesting.

RESISTANCE TRAINING

Resistance training is without a doubt the best exercise that you can do, but it is also the one that scares people the most. Which is why I'm starting with it!

Basically, resistance training is just any form of weight-bearing exercise. Effective resistance exercise doesn't have to be the extreme type that comes to mind when you think of people lifting big weights in the gym.

Standing up and sitting down in a chair is resistance exercise, with your body acting as a weight. Sitting on a bench, then holding onto the bench while lowering your bum to the floor and lifting yourself back up into the seated position is a resistance exercise for the backs of the arms. It can really be that simple. Your body is a weight and by using it, you will be doing the simplest and best resistance training possible.

No matter what age you are, how fit or unfit, resistance work will help to change your life. Here are some other reasons you should be doing resistance training:

Improving general health
If you have high cholesterol, a family history of cardiovascular disease or pretty much any medical condition, by doing some resistance training you will be reducing the effects and lowering your risk factors.

Building bone density
Your bones will weaken as you age and will get even weaker if you eat poorly and don't exercise. By doing resistance training, you are making them stronger, taking the pressure off your joints. If you have osteoporosis or arthritis, you especially need to do more weight-bearing exercise – it is far better for your bones and joints than supplements.

Speeding up your metabolism
Your metabolism – the rate at which you burn calories – is your body's inbuilt rev. counter. The higher it is, the more calories you burn on a daily basis. As you age, it slows down, unless you move more and eat better. Healthier people have high metabolic rates. Resistance training builds calorie-loving muscle.

Improving cellulite
Cellulite (fat stored densely under the surface of the skin, mainly on the hips and thighs, which makes the surface dimpled and puckered) is the bane of many women's lives and some men's too. Cleaning up your

The good news - or maybe the bad news, depending on your personality - is that just like with diet, there is no one-shot simple way of becoming fitter.

diet and deep-tissue massage will make a difference, but toning up with resistance training will have the most obvious visual impact. Also, as cellulite is reputed to inhibit the elimination of toxins from the body (they get trapped in the dense network of connective tissue and fat, which actually makes the cellulite look more pronounced), anything that improves circulation will help both cellulite and the skin's surface appearance.

Reducing your clothes size

It is great to measure your progress by weight and inches, but what better way to see the evidence than in the reduction of your dress or suit size? Remember, lean tissue takes up less space in the body than fat, so weight training will help you drop those clothes sizes more quickly than the other types of exercise – even more so if you combine it with another type. It won't make you bigger; it will give you tone and shape so that you not only look good, but feel good too!

Increasing strength

Being strong is in fashion at the moment, but it's also essential for life. The stronger you are, the more you reduce your chance of doing yourself damage, both in training and in everyday activities. That's important as you get older, when the body takes longer to recover from exertion or injury.

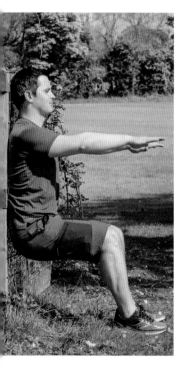

Improving posture

Our postures are getting worse. Because we sit and slouch all day, the muscles that help our posture don't get worked and they become weaker. Again, this is especially true as you get older. The weight of your head puts more and more pressure on your back and your core (the muscles around the midsection of your body). You become weak there and begin to slouch forward. You need to do resistance work to strengthen these muscles. This will not only relieve back pain, but also give you a flatter stomach, because when the body straightens up, your stomach is no longer pushed out from the body.

Reducing stress

By focusing on a resistance-exercise programme, you forget about your day. You put aside time for yourself, focus on the movements you are doing and, without thinking about them, you work out the stresses and strains of the day. You also release lots of hormones into the bloodstream, so you finish a session feeling calmer than you did when you started.

Resistance exercise will keep you firm, strong and lean, so no matter what other exercise you do, you should aim to get at least one resistance session into your week, working all the body parts. This is especially important as we get older, as it keeps the blood circulating around the body, improves hormone function and keeps your muscles strong and functional. In Chapter 20 (page 172) I will take you through three exercise series – grouped according to whether they focus on the upper or lower body or the core – that will keep you supplied with failsafe exercises for building your own resistance programme. You can do these at home for years to come!

Being strong is in fashion at the moment, but it's also essential for life.

CARDIOVASCULAR TRAINING

Cardiovascular training is probably the most accessible form of exercise there is. Any movement that gets your heart and lungs working – from walking to running, surfing to cycling – is cardiovascular. Once your heart rate increases and you get slightly out of breath, then you are doing it. And generally it can be done anywhere, which makes it easy for people to fit it into their lives.

The benefits of cardiovascular exercise include:

- **Fat burning:** Cardiovascular training, like any exercise, will help to burn calories. And if you're eating carefully and exercising consistently, you will start to burn the extra fat your body has stored.

- **Improvements in lung function:** Any exercise that gets you breathing heavily will mean that your lung capacity is being pushed to its limits and maintained. This will help your lungs to perform better, meaning that vital fresh oxygen is kept circulating around your body.

- **Stress release:** Any exercise that gets you out of your head and gets you moving will help to alleviate stress.

- **Hormone release:** The experts tell us that many beneficial hormones – including those affecting growth, appetite and mood – are released during strenuous exercise. You may have heard people talking about getting an 'endorphin high' or 'runner's high' from physical exertion – that's the feeling of wellbeing the body naturally produces after exercise. It's caused by a release of hormones – endorphins – that inhibit pain and lift mood. The effect is similar to morphine, so now you know why some people find exercise addictive!

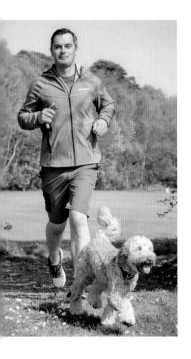

- **Muscle adaptation:** This means that your muscles learn to consume a greater amount of fuel and to do so more efficiently because you are exercising hard. It also means that as the muscles get stronger, they get used to longer, harder exercise.

Although it is so simple to do – or perhaps because it's so simple to do – cardiovascular exercise is generally the one where people make the biggest mistake, as they don't work hard enough. To get the very best value out of the time you spend working out, you have to exert yourself.

To check if you are working hard enough, do the 'talk test' – see if you are out of breath but just about able to hold a conversation or count to 10. If it's easy, you're not working hard enough. If you can't do it, you're overdoing things. You should never be fully out of breath when working out, as it means you are working too hard. Plus it's uncomfortable and may end up putting you off exercising.

The exception to the talk test is high-intensity interval training (HIIT), which has become very popular in the last few years. This method includes short bursts of very high-intensity activity where you do end up becoming breathless. While HIIT can be effective, it can also be off-putting to many people – most often those who most need to exercise. For that reason, I'm not going to use HIIT training in this book, as I want to make it as easy as possible for you to get healthy and fit.

No matter what your starting level of fitness, you can create a cardiovascular workout to suit your schedule that will make the most of the time you have and will help you burn the maximum number of calories in that time.

Gyms around the country are full of cardiovascular machines like steppers, rowers, treadmills and cross-trainers. These are your calorie-burning machines so if you are a member of a gym, use them, ideally in combination with a resistance-training programme. But if you're not in a gym, don't worry. You can do cardiovascular exercise outside in the open air, which is even better because generally you work harder when you don't have a machine doing some of the work.

Like every form of exercise, the key thing is to find an activity that you enjoy, that's accessible and that you can fit into your week. That way, it's more likely that you will keep it up and reap the rewards.

Like every form of exercise, the key thing is to find an activity that you enjoy, that's accessible and that you can fit into your week.

PASSIVE TRAINING

This is a somewhat overlooked form of exercise that can have huge benefits for every part of your body. Yoga, Pilates, t'ai chi, stretching, body balance and meditation are all types of passive exercise. I call these passive purely because they are often more chilled out than cardio or weights sessions. Though they may be less intense, they deliver fantastic benefits, especially as you age. They complement resistance and cardio work, improve flexibility, mobility and balance, and can make big differences to joint issues. Women tend to be great at this type of training while men, unfortunately, need to do more of it!

These exercises complement resistance and cardio work, improve flexibility, mobility and balance, and can make big differences to joint issues.

The feel-good factor from these is totally different to any other exercise high you may have come across before. You are still releasing endorphins, but you can feel very relaxed afterwards. So passive work is a super way to lower stress levels. Here are some of the other benefits:

- Reducing the risk of injury
- Reducing the risk of lower-back pain
- Reducing the risk of falls
- Reducing cholesterol and the risk of cardiovascular disease
- Reducing your medical bills
- Increasing your social network.

One of the main reasons that I love this type of exercise is that it often takes place in classes, so it gets you meeting up with like-minded people in your neighbourhood, which is particularly beneficial in rural areas and throughout the winter months.

Obviously, classes are a great way to get involved with this type of exercise, especially when you get a great teacher, but it isn't always possible to get to a class, or classes may be beyond your budget. In that case, you will find thousands of videos on YouTube, with different teachers and styles. Find one that you like and you can follow their sessions for free.

And if you can't get onto the internet, to get started straightaway, here are some of the stretches I use – both for myself and my clients.

Yoga upper-body bends

Start with your feet together, your hands directly above your head, palms together. Take a deep breath in and stretch your arms up to the sky, keeping your palms together. Now simply bend to the left and hold for 10 seconds. Come back to centre and bend to the right for 10 seconds. This is one set. Repeat for three sets. As your body begins to loosen up, you will find that you can bend further and further, but ease into it.

Shoulder rolls

The old-school classic, these are great to loosen up the shoulder joints and muscles. Start with your feet together and hands at the front of the body. Keeping the arms straight, roll the arms back in big circles for 10 rotations and then roll them forward for 10. This is one set. These should be done slowly, and you should aim to stretch the arms out as far as possible. Repeat for three sets.

Tricep stretch

The triceps at the back of the arm can get quite tight and often need a good stretch. Start with your feet together. Straighten the left arm above the head and the right arm straight down by your side. Now bend the left arm back behind the head and at the same time bend your right arm up towards your shoulder blades. Try to touch the hands in the centre of your back. If you can't touch your hands, don't worry – just hold a rolled-up towel between your hands and move your hands along it as far as you can. As you get more flexible, your hands will come closer together. Hold the stretch for 15 seconds and change hands. This is one set. Repeat for three sets.

The feel-good factor from passive training is totally different to any other exercise high you may have come across before. You are still releasing endorphins, but you can feel very relaxed afterwards.

Hip rolls

Time to get the hips moving and loosened out! Start with the feet shoulder-width apart and the back straight. Place your hands on your hips and roll the hips in big circles to the left for 10 rotations and then to the right for 10 rotations. That's one set. Go for three sets and try to make nice big circles.

Knee rolls

This is one of my favourite stretches and it's really simple. Stand with your legs together. Bend over gently and place your hands on the front of your knees. Now just roll your knees in a circular motion to the left for 10 rotations and then to the right for 10 rotations. That's one set. These should be easy and gentle; the idea is to loosen out the ligaments, tendons and muscles around the knee joint. Repeat for three sets.

Hamstring stretch

The hamstrings are a big muscle group at the back of the leg and if they become tight, it can lead to lower-back problems. With this stretch, stand with your feet together, back straight. Cross your right leg in front of your left, so that your right foot moves to the other side of your left foot. Now slowly lower your hands down towards your feet. Don't bounce on this one, just ease into it and stretch towards the toes as far as feels comfortable. Hold for 15 seconds and then swap legs. That's one set. Repeat for three sets.

Quad stretch

The quad is at the front of the legs and is a big muscle group. This is one of the simplest ways to stretch it out. Lie on your left side, propping your head up with your hand. Bend your right knee and bring your foot up towards your bum. Take your ankle in your right hand and hold it in this position for 15 seconds. Roll onto your right side and do the same with your left leg. When you've done both legs, that's one set. Repeat for three sets.

These stretches can be done on their own as a session or they can be used alongside more intensive forms of exercise.

These stretches can be done on their own as a session or they can be used alongside more intensive forms of exercise. The role of stretching before and after exercise is a topical subject at the moment. I do not favour using stretches for warming up. In my view, the body is cold at the start of a session and that increases the risk of injury. Not only is the body warmed up at the end of a session but, at that point, stretches can help to prevent soreness and to bring the heart rate down, which is important. If you want to stretch at the start of a session, aim to do a gentle warm-up first (even a little walking around), for around five minutes, and then do your stretches.

This routine can be a jumpstart to get you going and as you begin to feel the benefits, you can progress by researching new stretches and adding them to your repertoire. If you go online, you'll find some great routines on YouTube. And if you're scared of joining a class, becoming comfortable doing your own stretching routine might just give you the confidence to sign up!

18 A FITNESS PROGRAMME JUST FOR YOU

I am going to share with you a process I go through with all of my clients when they come in for their initial session. I believe that it is one of the keys to getting good results. This simple exercise only involves a pen and paper. It's about thinking everything through at the outset so that you build an intelligent exercise programme that suits you. Not only will it save you time and frustration, it will help you become fit and healthy and achieve your goals.

What you want to do is set out a four-to-six-week plan of action that includes the three elements I described in the last chapter – cardiovascular, resistance and stretching work. You won't do each element for an equal amount of time every day – for instance, on Day 1, you might plan a brisk walk at lunchtime and some specific resistance exercises that night in front of the TV, followed by a couple of stretches. The length and timing of the walk and the specific exercises should be listed in your plan. On Day 2 you could plan to get to the gym to do a session on the cardio machines in the morning (again, your plan will specify what machines and the time you will spend on each), followed by some stretching to cool down, and that'll be it for the day. On Day 3, you might know that you'll be out of town for work, so you plan to do a full resistance workout followed by stretching in your hotel room that night – each of the exercises you plan to do should be listed in your plan for the day. And so on. Over the course of a week, it should even out.

Organize yourself with a good thick notebook that will become your personal fitness journal where you write down all your plans, log your progress and jot down any observations. If you're happier working on a computer, open a document there. You can even send yourself your weekly exercise plan so you can access it wherever you are. To make your plan practical and easier to stick to, follow these principles when putting it together:

BE SPECIFIC

Remember that everyone is different and has different needs, so your programme should reflect this. If you have injuries, or weaknesses in certain areas, then take these into account. Maybe you need to strengthen your upper body more than your lower body. Or is your level of flexibility your weak area?

Draw a line down the middle of the page to make two columns. Write 'Strengths' at the top of one and 'Weaknesses' at the top of the other and underneath each heading, list the areas where you think you're doing well and the ones where you think there's room for improvement. And don't avoid the 'Strengths' column – even if you are very overweight and unfit, your body is still doing an amazing job for you. For starters, it's probably quite strong, so you may find yourself able to do more than you expect when it comes to resistance training.

Remember that everyone is different and has different needs, so your programme should reflect this.

WHAT'S YOUR MOTIVATION?

Now make a list of what you are aiming to get out of your fitness programme. This will act as your basis for creating it. If you work from here, you will get a real programme that will work for you and for your body. Some simple examples would be aiming to run 5km in under 30 minutes or losing 5cm from your waistline.

SET OUT YOUR TARGETS

You are building a programme for a reason and you'll want to be able to evaluate your progress. Of course, you will notice this by feeling and looking better, but it's great to be able to measure your progress too. Going further in the same amount time in your cardio session, lifting a heavier weight or completing more complicated exercises are all great examples of targets that could work for you.

You need to ensure that the programme you build is a fit for your life. While you are making changes to live a healthier life, that doesn't mean you can suddenly banish work and family responsibilities.

BE REALISTIC

What's your starting point and what's going on in your life? Are you building a programme for an Olympic athlete or for yourself? I often fall into this trap myself, building amazing sessions that would work great if I were a full-time athlete and had the time to recover and do nothing else!

You need to ensure that the programme you build is a fit for your life. While you are making changes to live a healthier life, that doesn't mean you can suddenly banish work and family responsibilities. You'll need to see what can be adjusted and what can't and has to be worked around. If you can't make your new programme work, it won't last long term and you will give up after a few weeks or so. You might even say it's 'impossible' for you to get fit when really it's about figuring out smaller and more realistic routines that you can integrate into your life.

And are you being too ambitious – for instance, aiming to lose too much weight in too short an amount of time so that the goal becomes a personal Everest and a millstone after a few weeks? Remember: modest and realistic goals that are reviewed and revised at regular intervals will help you to achieve your best and long-term change.

BE PREPARED

You don't need much stuff to start exercising, but it helps with motivation if you sort yourself out with the right gear. Here are some examples:

Resistance training: Trainers (*see* Chapter 21, page 206, for advice), workout gear, exercise mat, towel, hand weights (dumbbells), water, a plan to follow.

Running: Trainers (*see* Chapter 21, for advice), synthetic socks, a high-vis rain jacket, non-cotton-based clothing… and an event to aim for, such as a Parkrun!

Cycling: Bike, helmet, pump, tubes, cycling shorts, a high-vis rain jacket, water, fruit for a snack.

Hill-walking: A high-vis rain jacket, walking boots, backpack with phone, food and fluid, multiple layers to stay warm, a map (ensure you know the trail you are walking beforehand and tell someone where you are heading if going alone).

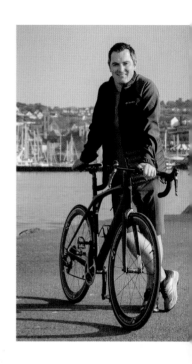

GIVE YOURSELF A TIMEFRAME

Set a time limit on this plan and aim to change the plan every four to six weeks. Your body adapts to changes in routine and movement quite quickly. If you try to do the same exercise at the same effort level again and again, it becomes too easy for the body and you won't get the results that you want. But if you keep changing your workouts, you will get ongoing change in your body. This will mean you have to change your programme a lot and on an ongoing basis. While for some of you this might seem a little tiresome – some people, I know, are creatures of habit! – you will build up a big repertoire and understanding of various exercises, and in time

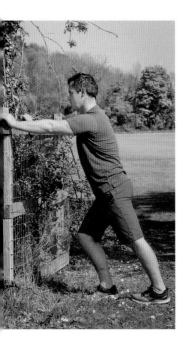

making changes every month or so won't feel like a big deal. You'll start to do it intuitively, depending on what's going on with your body.

DON'T FORGET ABOUT WARMING UP AND COOLING DOWN

No matter what exercises you put in your plan, make sure to schedule time to warm up at the start and cool down at the end of every session. The purpose of warming up and cooling down is to avoid injury, keeping you away from the physiotherapist and keeping you healthy for longer. It's particularly important to cool down at the end of a session, as it will help you avoid muscle soreness in the days following your workout.

Generally, I use a five-minute warm-up and a five-minute cool-down routine with my clients. This allows the muscles to warm up safely and cool down nicely, letting the blood vessels contract slowly. An ideal warm-up is walking on the spot, walking upstairs or even a quick walk around the block. And the stretches I described in the previous chapter are perfect for your cool-down.

LISTEN TO YOUR BODY

If you feel any pain or soreness when you make particular moves, stop immediately. If the soreness persists or is always there when you move in a particular way, book an appointment with a physiotherapist or your GP and get it checked out. You will injure yourself and sabotage your plans if you persist in exercising when you are in pain. Men in particular tend to want to keep going regardless. That is simply stupid. Looking after yourself properly when you are injured is a positive thing to do for your body and your long-term health. If you need to rest a particular part of your body, a physiotherapist or fitness instructor will be able to advise you on other things you can do to work around the problem and stay as fit as you realistically can until things improve. Warming up and cooling down properly and stretching regularly will help you avoid injuries. Chapter 22 (page 210) covers back health and dealing with injuries.

ON THE SEVENTH DAY, REST!

Often when you start exercising, you go for it with the gusto of a January gym member – training hard and really pushing the body. This often leads to overtraining, meaning that you've pushed your body beyond its capacity for repair and you are injured or in danger of becoming injured.

The easiest way to avoid overtraining is by allowing at least one day per week when you put your feet up and stay away from exercise. This day will give your muscles time to repair themselves and your mind time to recover, keeping you fresh for the following week's workouts. Rest – and especially sleep – is the body's best way to recover, so aim to get the best quality of sleep that you can. (I have some more information about sleep in Chapter 25, page 224.)

If you keep all these elements in mind as you put together a programme, you will ensure that you get the results you want. And when you hit your targets, give yourself a clap on the back and treat yourself to something nice!

And when you hit your targets, give yourself a clap on the back and treat yourself to something nice!

19 BUILDING YOUR OWN STRENGTH PROGRAMME

Earlier, I said that weight-bearing exercise is the best type you can do. Not only that, it's also very simple to put together your own weight-training plan that you can do at home in your own time, with no special equipment needed apart from a set of weights.

You can get a simple pair of inexpensive hand weights, or dumbbells, from the sports section of a department store, a sports shop, Argos or online. For women, a good starting weight is 2kg. Men might want to start at 3kg. As you get fitter and stronger, you may need to go up a weight. If you can't get weights, just use a bottle of water, but be careful how you grip it – you don't want to strain your wrist.

In this chapter, I'm sharing a series of exercises for the three main body segments – lower body, upper body and core – that will give you enough options to give you months and months of possible training combinations. It's a pick and mix of exercises that will make a big change to your health and your body. Here's how to put your plan together:

1 Generally try to pick TWO exercises per body segment, but if you're really short on time, don't worry – any is better than none.

2 To help you choose, I have colour coded each exercise for three different levels of fitness: beginner, intermediate or advanced.

3 Warm up for five minutes.

4 Complete one, two or three sets of 15 to 20 repetitions.

5 Cool down for five minutes.

Here is a table that will help you put together four programmes to get you going. Simply choose the exercises from each category and fill them in on the table. Add in your warm-up and cool-down and you're good to go. Once you get into the exercise, you'll be coming up with new programmes all the time.

	PROGRAMME 1	PROGRAMME 2	PROGRAMME 3	PROGRAMME 4
WARM UP				
LOWER 1				
LOWER 2				
UPPER 1				
UPPER 2				
CORE 1				
CORE 2				
COOL DOWN				

When you are starting out, I would recommend one set of 20 repetitions of the exercises for the first week (except where I specify a different number of reps) and then build it up from there. As you get stronger, you can build up to two and then three sets. Ideally you should aim not to be too sore after your session, so by building it up slowly, you will be taking a much safer approach, reducing the risk of injury.

From time to time in the exercises, I remind you to keep your core engaged. What this means is that the muscles around your torso – your core – are doing their work to support your back. You can make sure your core is engaged by checking that you're not slumping, your head is erect (i.e. looking straight ahead rather than down) and your back is straight (but not rigid), your shoulders are relaxed and not tensed up and, if you can, you should pull your belly button in towards your spine as you go through each exercise, just like holding in your tummy for a photograph!

Aim to change your programme after you can do three sets comfortably, building up your fitness levels over four weeks or so, and taking on the harder exercises and/or using heavier weights.

In the pages that follow, the various lower, upper and core exercises are demonstrated by my neighbours Natalie and Paul, pictured with me on the facing page. They are both keen exercisers but neither is a fitness professional. (The dog, Sophie, also got in on the fun!)

Ideally you should aim not to be too sore after your session, so by building it up slowly, you will be taking a much safer approach, reducing the risk of injury.

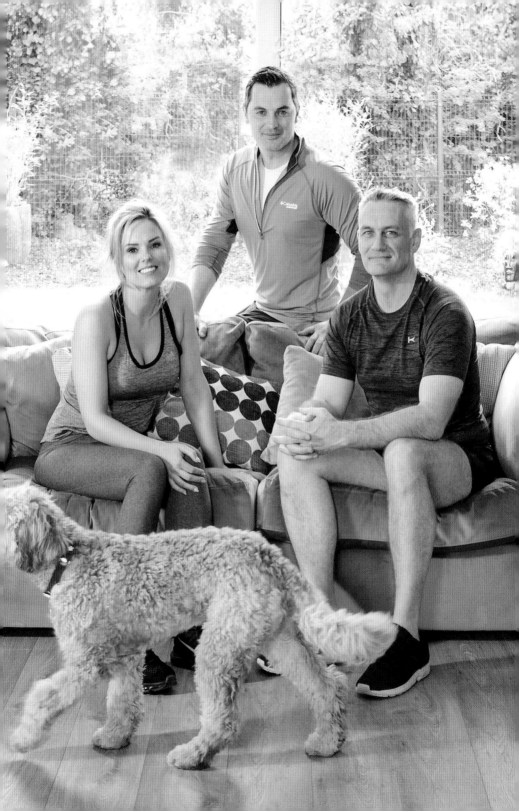

LOWER-BODY EXERCISES

SIDE LEG RAISE

Lie on your side on the floor for this one. Ensure all of your joints are in one line: your ankles, knees, hips and shoulders. Keeping your leg straight, flex your foot so that your toes point towards your face and then raise your leg as far as feels comfortable and lower it back down. If you want to make it harder, you can simply hold your leg in the air for 30 seconds at the end of your 20 reps. Lie on your other side and repeat. This is one set.

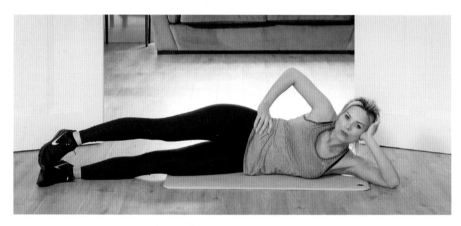

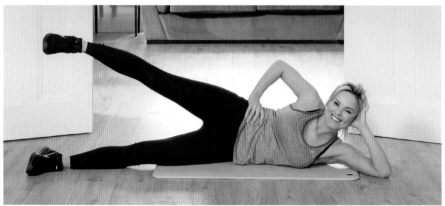

SKI SQUAT

●●

A classic exercise that will help to improve leg strength for anyone of any age, so you have no excuses! Stand with your back against a wall, feet shoulder-width apart out in front of you about two feet from the wall. Now lower your body down until your thighs are parallel to the floor. Ensure your knees never extend over your toes. Hold for as long as you can. You should be able to hold this position for at least 30 seconds.

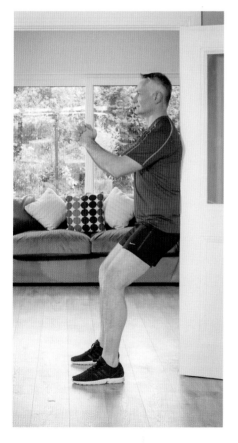
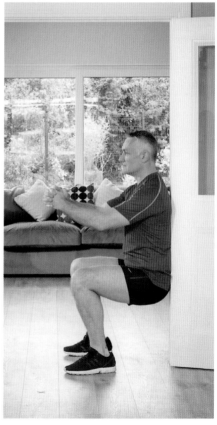

LUNGE

Start with your feet together and hands on your hips. Take a big step forward on your left foot and bend your right knee towards the floor. Stand up straight. Repeat 20 times on the left leg and then 20 times on the right.

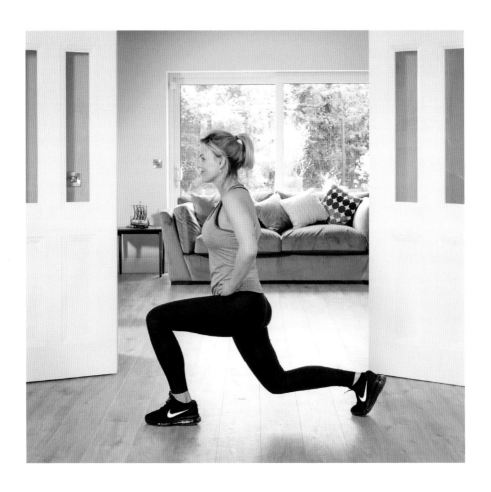

WIDE FOOT SQUAT

● ● ●

This has always been one of my favourite exercises. Start with your feet wider than shoulder-width apart, with your toes pointing away from the body and your hands crossed at shoulder level in front of the body. Now gently lower your bum down towards the floor until you get to a seating position and hold. This is the starting position. From here, simply pulse your bum up and down by about three inches.

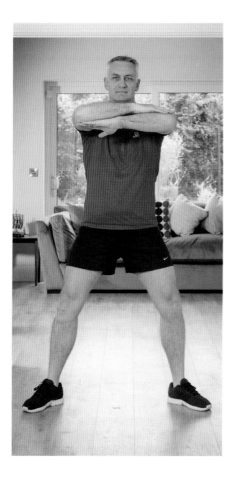

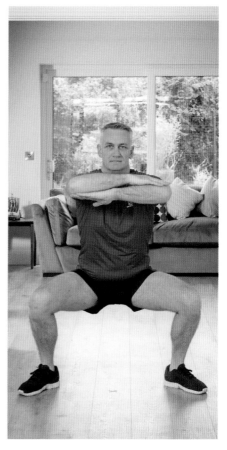

SUMO SQUAT

A great exercise for the inside of the legs and outside of the bum too. Start with your feet wider than shoulder-width apart, with your hands on your hips. Simply squat down and as you begin to stand up, roll the right leg in a circular motion to the right and then squat again. Stay on the right side for 20 reps and then repeat on the left.

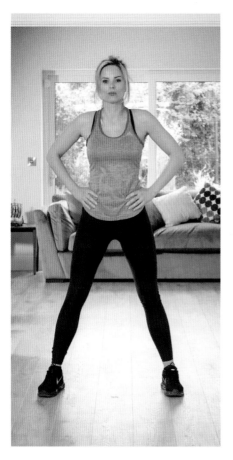
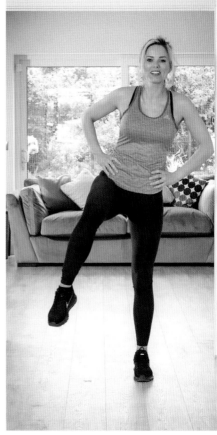

SQUAT

● ● ●

Start with your feet shoulder-width apart and your hands crossed at shoulder level in front of the body. Simply bend your knees and lower your bum as low as feels comfortable, aiming to push through your heels on the way down. Then come back to standing. Repeat 20 times.

HALF SQUAT

● ●

A simple yet demanding addition to the full squat. This is a great way to put your legs through a harder workout without having to add weight. For the exercise, start in your usual squat position. Now, when you squat down, aim to go all the way down to the seated position but only return halfway up, then lower back down again. Repeat 20 times.

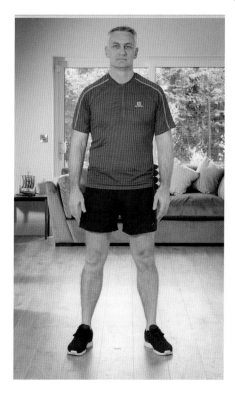
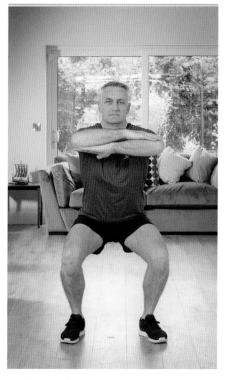

STEP UP

This can be done on a low wall or park bench and is great for all the muscles of the lower body. Stand in front of the wall or bench with your collarbone wide and shoulders and back straight, with your hands on your hips. Simply step up onto the bench/wall with the right leg 20 times, then repeat with the left leg. If it's too easy, just look for a higher bench.

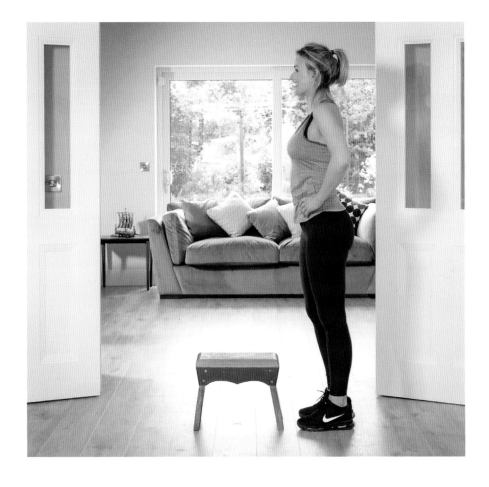

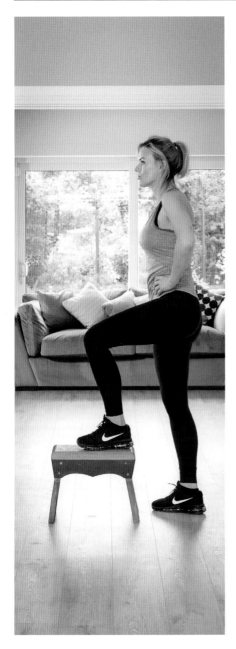
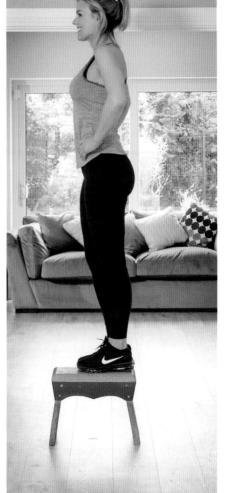

JUMP SQUAT

This exercise is a little tougher than most, but you might be ready for it by about Week 5! It's simple enough to do: start with your feet shoulder-width apart. Now bend down, keeping your back straight and arms by your sides, and tap your ankles with your fingers and then jump as high as you can.

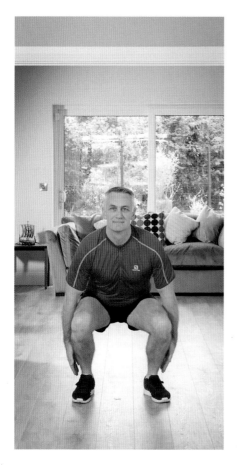
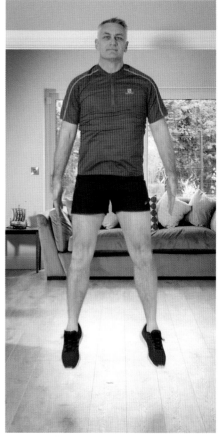

UPPER-BODY EXERCISES

FRONT RAISE

For this exercise, you will need your weights. Start with your feet shoulder-width apart and hold your weights to the front of your body at hip level. Keeping your arms straight, knuckles facing away from the body and your back straight, raise the weights to eye level and return to hip level. Repeat 20 times.

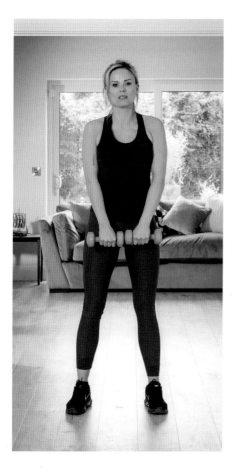
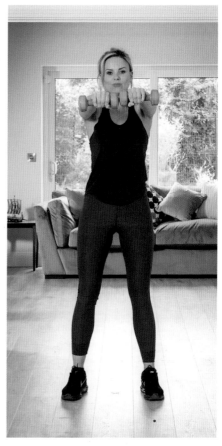

MILITARY PRESS

One of the classics! Begin with your feet shoulder-width apart, your back straight and your core muscles engaged. Start with your arms bent, holding your weights at shoulder level. Straighten your arms up towards the ceiling, pressing the weight up. (Ideally your arms will be a little straighter than Paul's are in the photograph.) Return to the starting position, with the weights back at shoulder level. Repeat 20 times.

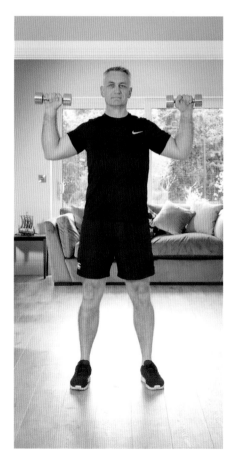
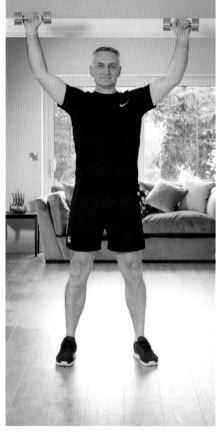

BICEP CURL

The classic exercise for your biceps at the front of your arms. Start with your feet shoulder-width apart, arms by your sides, holding your weights in both hands. Keep your elbows glued to the side of your waist and lift the weights up to your shoulder. Return to the starting position. Repeat 20 times. As always, keep your back straight and your core engaged throughout this exercise.

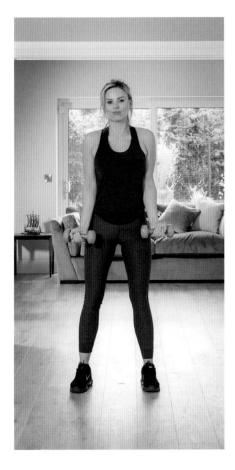

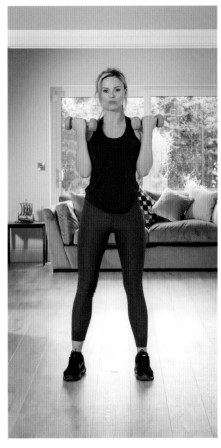

TRICEP DIP

One of my favourite exercises, as it's so easy to do and so good for your upper body. Start by sitting on a bench, stairs or stable chair. Place your feet out in front of you, keeping your arms by your sides, hands curled around the front edge of the bench/chair. Now simply bend the elbows and lower your bum towards the floor, making sure to keep your bum/back close to the bench/chair. If it's too easy, move your legs further away, and if it's too hard, bring your legs closer to you. Repeat 20 times.

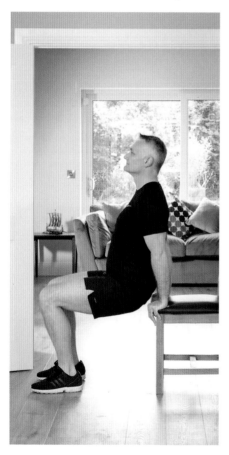
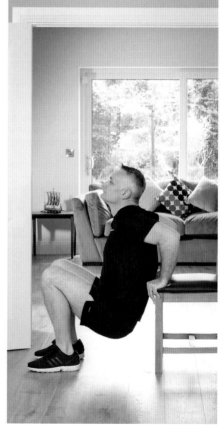

SIDE LATERAL RAISE

Start with your feet shoulder-width apart, arms straight down by your sides, holding your weights. Raise your straight arms up and out from your body so that you form a T-shape. Return them to the starting position. Repeat 20 times. The important thing is to ensure that your shoulders are pulled back – this engages the deltoid muscle in your shoulder and helps to improve your posture and prevent rounded shoulders.

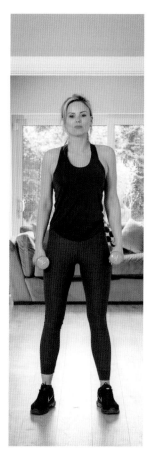

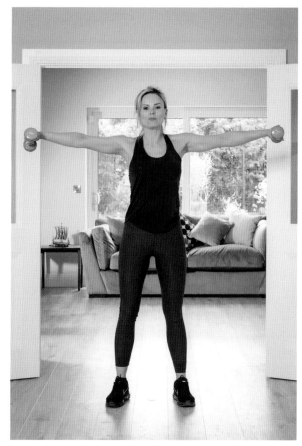

SHOULDER CIRCLE

This is one of my favourite exercises for your shoulders. There are four parts to it:

1 Start with your feet shoulder-width apart, holding the weights by your sides, wrists facing forwards. Now simply complete a circle for 10 reps by moving your arms from your sides to above your head, keeping your arms straight.

2 Standing in the same position, still holding the weights, move your arms so that they are straight out at right angles from your shoulders (so your body is in a T-position). Raise your arms so they meet above your head and return back to shoulder level.

3 For the third part, standing in the same position and still holding the weights, start with your arms straight down by your sides, the weights at hip level. Raise your arms straight out in front of you to shoulder height and then return them back down to your sides.

4 For the final part, simply go back to the full circle for 10 reps. Be careful not to arch your back, especially for these, as you will be more tired.

The four elements here make up one set.

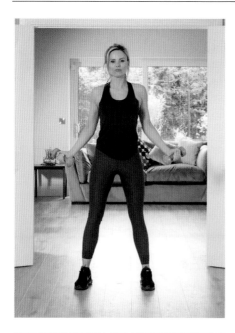

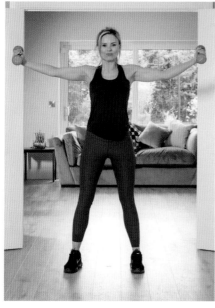

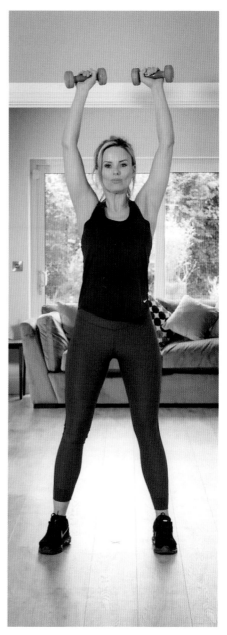

REVERSE PRESS

A great exercise for your shoulders and back. Start with your feet shoulder-width apart, holding your weights at the top of your chest, with your elbows tucked loosely by your sides. Keeping your back straight, simply extend the weights up towards the ceiling and return to the top of your chest. Repeat 20 times.

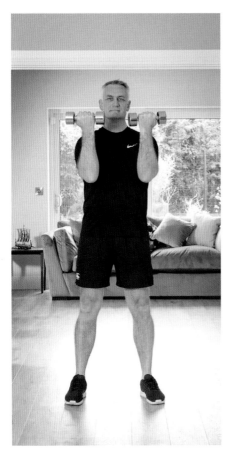
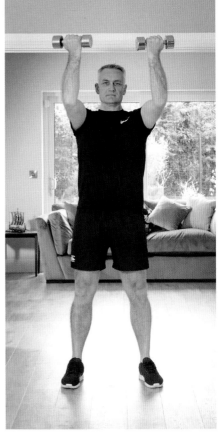

PRESS UP

Another classic that's great for the upper body and so easy to do. Lie on the floor, face down. Place your hands either side of your shoulders and a little out from your shoulders. Feet together. Raise yourself up on your arms. Start with arms straight and back straight so that your hips are in a straight line with your shoulders. Now bend at the elbows and lower your chest towards the floor, still keeping your back straight. You can also do this with your knees on the floor; just ensure there is a straight line from your shoulders to your hips if you do. Repeat 20 times.

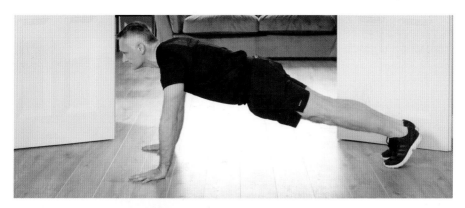

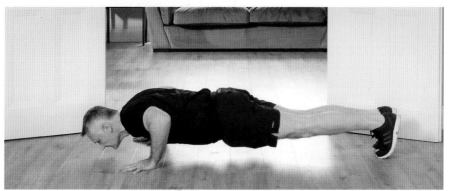

CORE EXERCISES

HANDS-ON-KNEES SIT-UP

Start by lying on the floor, knees bent and feet shoulder-width apart. Place your hands on the front of your thighs, making sure your neck is relaxed. Now simply move your hands up towards your knees. As you do, your upper body will naturally lift up off the floor. Return your hands back to their starting position. As you do this exercise, keep your eyes looking towards a point on the ceiling to take the pressure off your neck. Repeat 20 times.

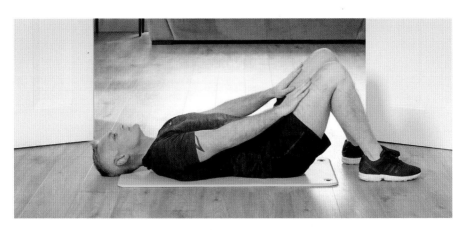

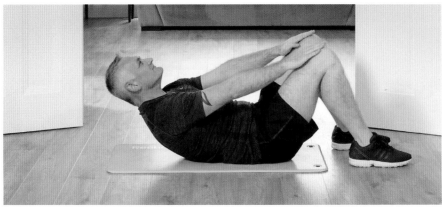

LEG HOLDS

I have always loved this exercise. Start by lying on your back, knees bent and feet together. Now raise your feet off the floor so that your calves are parallel to the floor. Hold for as long as you can. As you get stronger you will be able to hold it for longer.

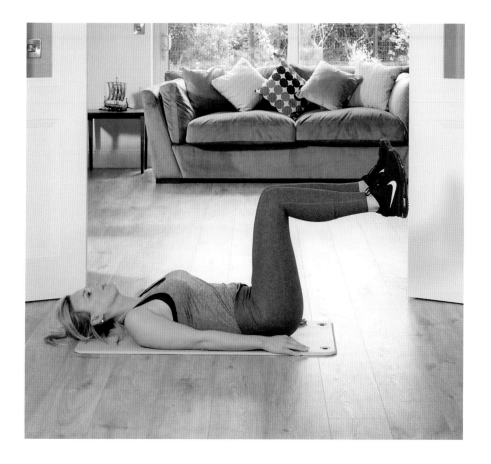

ANKLE TAPS

An old-school classic that's really good for your waistline. Start by lying on your back, knees bent and feet together. Keep your hands by your sides and then, reaching down slightly on your right side, simply tap your right ankle with your right hand. Go back to the starting position and then reach down and tap your left ankle with your left hand. When you have done both the right and left that's one rep – repeat for 20. Keep your neck relaxed and if you have any neck pain stop straight away.

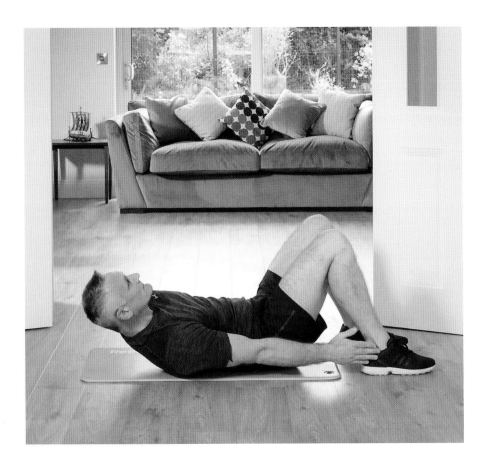

KNEE TO CHEST

●●

Start by lying on the floor with your hands under your bum, palms facing the floor. Bring your knees in towards your chest and then push your legs away from your body, without resting them on the floor. Ensure your lower back is always flat on the floor and not arching up. The lower you go with your feet the more pressure there will be on your lower back. Stop if you feel any lower-back pain.

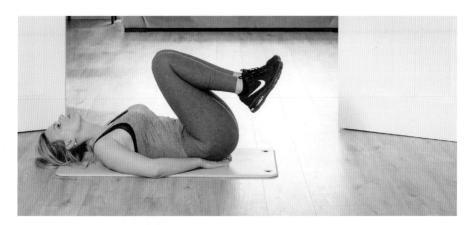

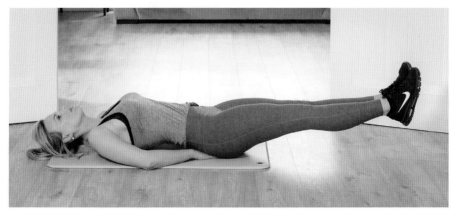

STRAIGHT-ARM PLANK

A simple but great exercise for the middle part of the body. It starts the same way as a press-up. Lie on the floor, face down. Place your hands either side of your shoulders and a little out from your shoulders. Feet together. Raise yourself up on straight arms. You are going to hold here for as long as you can. Aim for 30 seconds as an initial goal and then try to build it up. Pull your stomach in towards your spine while holding the position and keeping your back straight.

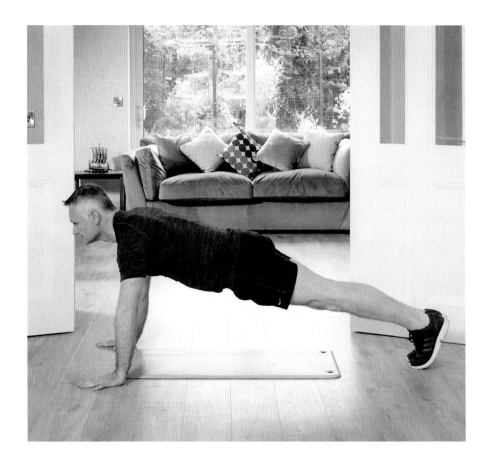

GLUTE BRIDGE

One of my favourite exercises for working the bum muscles! Start by lying on the floor on your back. Now bend your knees, with your feet shoulder-width apart, and place your hands down by your sides. Push your pelvis up to the ceiling and squeeze your bum as you do. Hold for five seconds, then return to the floor. Repeat for 20.

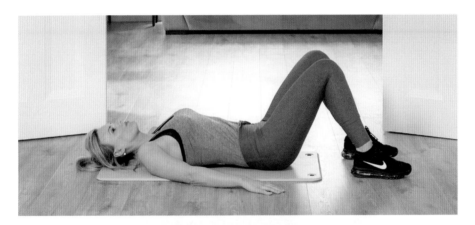

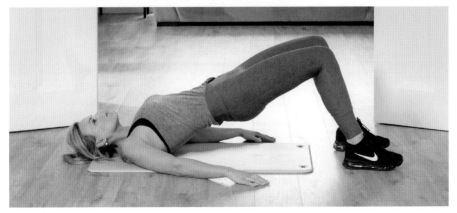

AB CRISS-CROSSER

Start by lying on the floor with your hands under your bum, palms to the floor. Raise your legs to a 45-degree angle off the floor and keep them straight. Cross one leg over the other and keep going, alternating legs for 20 reps. Each crossover counts as one rep. The lower the legs go the harder it gets.

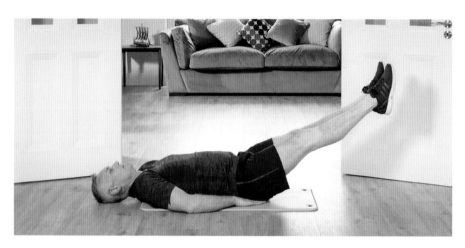

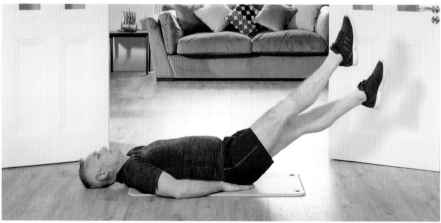

STRAIGHT LEG RAISES

Start by lying on the floor with your hands under your bum, palms facing the floor. Lift your legs to the 45-degree position. Lower one leg and raise the other. Simply alternate for 20 reps. If it's hard on your back then don't go quite so low on the way down.

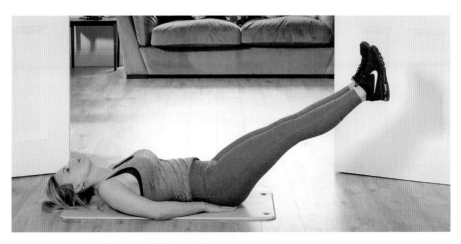

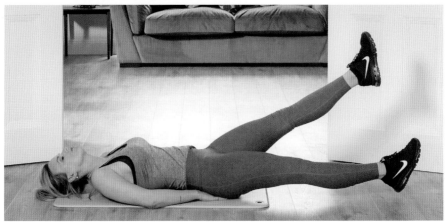

SIDE PLANK

This can be done in conjunction with the normal plank or on its own. For the side plank, begin on your right side, propping up your body with your forearm (your elbow should be under your shoulder) and with your shoulders, hips, knees and ankles in a straight line. Simply raise your hips off the floor, holding the straight line of your body, and hold the position for a long as you can. Make sure you are looking forward, not down at your body. Engage your core by pulling your bellybutton in towards your spine. You can use your left hand to stabilize the body if you need to. Repeat on the left side.

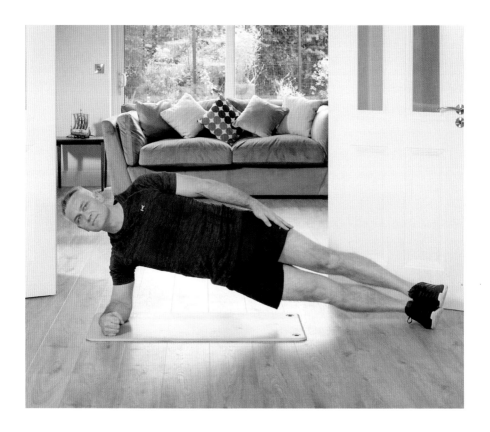

PLANK

This is great for the core and centre of the body. Just aim to do it for as long as you feel is challenging. (Why not have a competition with your family to see who can last the longest?) Lie face down on the floor. Start with your feet together, knees and elbows on the floor, with your elbows directly under your shoulders. Raise your body off the floor, pulling your bellybutton in towards your spine, and hold. Keep your back straight, your hips in line with your shoulders, and make sure you are looking down, not up, to ensure your head is in line with your body and to avoid neck strain.

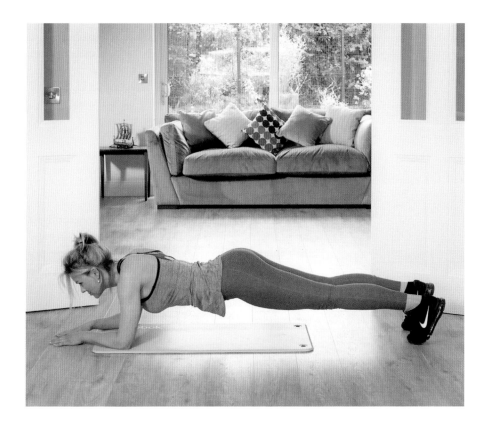

EFFORT LEVELS

When you exercise, your body does many cool things. It changes its shape. It uses fuel in the form of fat, carbs or protein. It releases hormones that make you feel better and repair your muscles. It slows down the ageing process. All of these things vary depending on how hard you work. There are three effort levels that you can work to:

Easy: If you are exercising and never getting out of breath, never breaking a sweat and never feeling that you have worked hard then, to be honest, it's of very little benefit in terms of losing weight or increasing your fitness level. Walking and swimming are probably the two exercises that a lot of people do and commonly don't see results. I see this with new clients all the time. There are some benefits, of course, to walking or swimming at a relaxed pace – moving, getting out into the fresh air, meeting people – but usually the body just isn't getting pushed enough for these to be really transformative.

The reality is that most of us are busy and want to get the most out of exercising. So it's a pity not to get a return on the time invested.

Hard: I classify hard exercise as when you get fully out of breath. This is what happens when you do high-intensity interval training (HIIT) or other types that push you to your max. There is no doubt that you get the most benefits here in terms of stress relief, hormone release and body change, and some people love to work at this level of intensity. But for many others, it is very uncomfortable and can be a scary experience. And if you don't like something, it doesn't have any place in your health plans because it simply won't last.

Moderately hard: This is the mid-point between the two. Moderately hard is hard enough that you feel you have had a workout, but not so hard that it becomes a barrier to exercise. You are still getting the hormone release, the stress benefits and the fat-burning properties, but it is doable, enjoyable and rewarding.

Working moderately hard is working at roughly 70 per cent of your heart-rate maximum. You can measure this by using a heart-rate monitor. However, there is a far simpler way of assessing how hard you are working – and that's by using the 'talk test' that I mentioned in Chapter 18 (page 160). Remember, this simply means that when you are exercising, you must be out of breath but still just about able to hold a conversation or count to 10.

The beauty of the talk test is that it's easy to do and it's free, so no matter what exercise you do, you will be able to perform to the level of intensity that gives you the greatest benefits. And as you get fitter, you will have to work harder to hit your talk-test point, so your results won't plateau as they normally do. If you take nothing else from this book, I hope this will be a tool that you will be able to use for the rest of your exercising life!

The reality is that most of us are busy and want to get the most out of exercising. So it's a pity not to get a return on the time invested.

20 GET RUNNING!

As those of you who are familiar with me from TV will know, I'm a big fan of running! It's one of the best cardiovascular exercises you can do. Anyone of any age or any size can learn how to run – it's simple and easy to do. Take a look at the tips below and get yourself started.

1 SET A GOAL

No matter how big or small, having a goal will keep you focused and keep you working. And when you reach your goal it builds your confidence in working towards your next goal.

Pick a 5km, a 10km or even a marathon and put it in the diary. Work out what the interim goals are to make sure you're ready for the big day. These goals, although simple, will be one of the key factors in keeping you moving when the going gets tough. Don't forget to make your goals visual – put them on the fridge, in your diary or at your desk, anywhere you can see them! The more you can see them, the greater the chance you will stick to them.

2 RUNNING SHOES

It is essential to ensure that your feet are in the best running shoes possible, and that doesn't necessarily mean the most expensive. One of my key recommendations to any runner – beginner or otherwise – is to get a gait analysis done before you start training. Gait analysis just checks how you walk or run to ensure that you are getting into the best trainers to suit your foot type. Amphibian King is the company that I recommend for this and they have five stores nationwide that offer this service.

Most people, if they are running on a regular basis, should look at changing their running shoes every four to six months. (If you are walking regularly rather than running, then you should be getting a little longer wear out of them.) Remember to keep checking your trainers every month, ensuring that the absorption system is firm and not too soft.

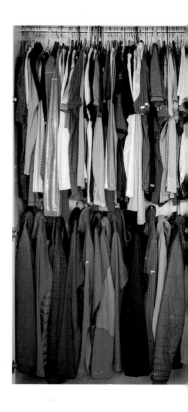

3 DRI-FIT GEAR

This is every athlete's best friend – clothing that works to eliminate sweat and will help keep you as dry as possible. All sports brands use some form of dri-fit fabric now, so stock up. Avoid cotton clothing as this holds on to water, becomes heavy and uncomfortable and can increase the risk of chafing or blisters.

4 BLISTERS

Getting blisters is one of the most annoying parts of starting to run. If you have soft feet then increase the amount of time you spend walking around barefoot as this will naturally toughen your feet really quickly. With new running shoes, only wear them for short runs for the first week or two and then gradually increase your distance in them. It is amazing how even experienced runners forget this rule!

If you find that you are still getting chafing, apply a little Vaseline to the affected areas. Rub it in deeply and this should solve the problem. The final tip is to wear the right socks – made from synthetic fabrics, as 1000 Mile socks are – as these will help reduce sweat around your feet and let them breathe better.

5 MAKE YOUR RUN A PART OF YOUR DAY

Why not try to run on your lunch break, or on the way home from work? This reduces the amount of excuses you can make to get out of doing your session and takes pressure off trying to shoehorn in time for a run when you may be rushing in the morning or busy at night.

6 QUALITY NOT QUANTITY

Don't just run for the sake of getting the miles in. If your body is tired then get some rest instead; it will make all the difference, not just to the run, but to the feel-good factor you get after it. Aim to do quality runs as opposed to just running because you feel you have to.

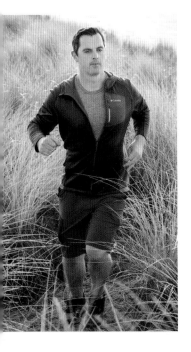

7 OVERTRAINING

Overtraining means you are pushing your body too hard. Symptoms such as tiredness, lack of appetite, high heart rates, illness and being on bad form are indicators of overtraining. The biggest indicator is if you go out for an easy session and it feels extremely hard. If this happens then simply head for home, put your feet up and recover. Rest is the best way to recover until you feel back to your normal self.

8 ENJOY DOWNTIME

You should have at least one day a week when you rest and relax, doing no exercise or work, and just let the mind unwind. By doing this you, will help to keep your stress levels to a minimum. Do something that you enjoy and leave your mind free to roam and come up with new ideas that you might not otherwise have come up with!

9 MOUNTAINS AND HILLS

One of the best and most fun ways to improve your road running is to head for the hills and get running in the mountains. It's not for the beginner, but as you begin to run more, hills and mountains provide a great way to strengthen your body and increase your fitness pretty quickly. It will build calf muscles and leg power that you previously thought unachievable. When you come back to run on the roads, you will see just how much faster you have become. There is also the Irish Mountain Running Association (www.imra.ie), which has races all year round.

Sometimes it can be hard to do it alone, so why not enlist your friends or colleagues at work?

10 GET YOUR FRIENDS INVOLVED

Sometimes it can be hard to do it alone, so why not enlist your friends or colleagues at work? Why not get a group together once or twice a week to run together? You could have a competition to see who exercises the most or loses the most weight, with a small prize at the end of the month. This is something that my friends and I do all the time, and it makes such a difference to your motivation!

21 MANAGING OBSTACLES TO GETTING FITTER AND HEALTHIER

There are a number of genuine reasons why sticking to your health and fitness plans might be challenging. Some of these are one-off – like injury – and others, such as back pain or PMS, can flare up regularly. Either way, there are measures you can take to deal with each of these.

WHAT TO DO ABOUT AN INJURY

Everyone should know the basics of managing injuries so that if you or one of your family or friends gets injured, you know exactly how to manage it. (I'd add that, regardless of your level of fitness, I am not at all worried about you getting injured following any of the plans in this book if you follow the instructions carefully.) The first-aid protocol for dealing with a soft-tissue injury, such as an ankle or knee sprain, is known by the acronym RICE:

Rest: The more movement you place upon an injured area, the worse the injury may become, so rest is essential to protect the injured muscle, tendon or ligament from further damage. If you feel an injury coming on then it's crucial to stop straight away.

Ice: Ice provides short-term pain relief and also limits swelling by reducing blood flow to the injured area. When icing an injury, choose either a cold pack, crushed ice wrapped in a plastic bag and then in a tea towel or a bag of frozen peas, also wrapped in a tea towel. Do not apply ice directly onto the skin. Never leave ice on an injury for more than 20 minutes at a time, as you can damage the skin with ice burn. And take the ice pack off the skin every two minutes and check for soreness or extreme redness, as these can be signs of ice burn. Another great tip for reducing swelling is arnica cream or arnica tablets.

Compression: This means wrapping the area of the injury to limit and reduce swelling, which may delay healing. Some people also experience pain relief from compression. You can apply the compression yourself or pick up a support from your local chemist. The wrapping should be snug but not tight. If it is too tight, you will be reducing blood flow to the injured area, which will slow down recovery. If you feel throbbing, remove the bandage and re-wrap the area so the bandage is a little looser.

Elevation: Elevating an injury helps control swelling by improving circulation to the area. It's most effective when the injured area is raised above the level of the heart. So, if you injure an ankle, try lying on your bed with your foot propped up on one or two pillows to get the leg elevated and the blood flowing back towards the body. If it's an arm injury then try to keep the arm up above chest level, even in small intervals, as it will reduce initial swelling quite quickly.

There are a number of genuine reasons why sticking to your health and fitness plans might be challenging.

After a day or two of RICE treatment, many sprains, strains or other injuries will begin to heal and get better. But if your pain or swelling does not decrease after 48 hours, make an appointment to see your GP or chartered physiotherapist, or go straight to the local hospital emergency department or Swiftcare clinic if you are really worried.

WHAT TO DO ABOUT BACK PAIN

Back issues and back pain are one of the most common complaints I come across when screening new clients or giving talks. This is a subject I am very familiar with – I have a curvature in my spine, my dad had two discs taken out and my mum has a twisted pelvis, so between us as a family we have accumulated quite a bit of experience in dealing with the back! I am not a physiotherapist and will always direct people to a physio when required, but I love working with clients on their back issues. From my years of experience, I know there are some simple things you can do to both reduce your risk of back issues and also help alleviate the pain when it flares up.

Movement: The first thing to remember is that backs need movement – normally low-intensity movement such as walking or swimming if you're having back pain. Fast walking is one of my favourite ways to loosen out a bad back. Walk on a flat route rather than uneven or hilly ground. Unless advised to do so, sitting for long periods of time is never good for your back; it will tend to stiffen up and just get worse.

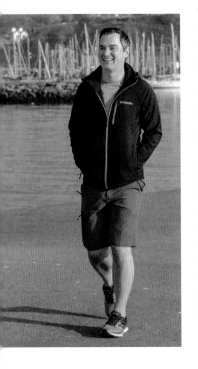

Flexibility: The next thing to look at is your level of flexibility. Tight hamstrings and bad backs always go together. Your hamstrings are the muscles at the backs of your legs and poor flexibility here will dramatically increase your risk of back issues. You can test your hamstring flexibility by sitting on the floor, with your feet together, legs straight out in front of you. Simply raise your hands in the air and lower them down, trying to touch your toes. How far can you get? In an ideal world, you should be able to touch your toes or get close to them along the shin. You can use a towel to help you improve this: wrap it around your feet and hold either end with your hands. Creep your hands along the towel gently to bring yourself further forward and give yourself a stretch. Try the hamstring stretch in Chapter 18 too (page 164).

Posture: Back problems and poor posture very often go together. We are designed to stand up straight. Yet between work, lack of activity and watching a lot of TV, people have worse posture than ever. I have two tips for improving posture. First, pull your belly button in towards your spine when sitting/ standing/walking – this will naturally force you to straighten up and strengthen your abdominal muscles. Second, don't sit or stand for long periods of time with both feet flat on the ground. By doing this, you are naturally placing more pressure on your lower back. Instead, get a book or box about 10cm in height and place one foot on this during the day, randomly alternating your feet. You will be surprised at the difference it makes!

Strength: Do some resistance training! Back issues can also be down to lack of strength in different parts of the body, particularly the core. Core muscles play a vital role in supporting your back. Resistance training is the obvious way to improve that. The exercises in Chapter 20 (page 172) are all perfect ways to get some more weight-bearing exercise into your day.

Massage: Massage can be a great way to loosen out a tight back. But do a bit of homework first – many of the massages offered in beauty salons and spas won't get stuck into the right muscle groups. Ideally, go for a sports massage, deep-tissue massage or a Ki Massage; all of these are great for your muscles, your circulation and your recovery too.

From my years of experience, I know there are some simple things you can do to both reduce your risk of back issues and also help alleviate the pain when it flares up.

WHAT TO DO ABOUT PMS

Women have an increased risk of water retention and temporary weight gain during the run-up to a period, mainly due to the changes in their hormone levels. In most women, the excess fluid can last for a few days, but it is not uncommon for the effects to last a lot longer. While monthly weight gain associated with the menstrual cycle is fluid not fat, it can be part of a range of symptoms that affect you at this time, including:

- swelling of breasts, abdomen, ankles and fingers
- headaches and even migraines
- back pain
- fatigue
- cramping

Hormones – alone or in combination with other body chemicals – can cause the body to swell due to increased fluid retention. This causes a bloated, heavy feeling for a week to 10 days before your period. The hormone progesterone reduces just before a period. Progesterone is involved in sodium regulation and is a natural diuretic so when it falls, you excrete less water through urination.

I have discussed these symptoms with so many of my female clients and I have seen the changes that being fit can have on their PMS symptoms. There is no doubt a link between your health and the duration of the PMS effects. The good news is that you can reduce the amount of fluid you retain and reduce the effects of your period dramatically by getting healthier and using the diet and fitness information in this book. Some other tips to target PMS symptoms include:

Sodium: Limit your sodium intake to around 500mg, or 0.5g, a day. That's about a quarter of a teaspoon, so very little. Sodium is a definite cause of fluid retention, so reduce or cut out salt in your diet and you will see a dramatic difference in your fluid-retention levels pretty much straight away. Avoid processed foods, which can have a lot of added salt. Breakfast cereals are surprisingly high in sodium, so check out the label on your favourite. Focus on eating plenty of fresh fruit and vegetables. Be very sparing when adding salt when cooking and use only good sea salt (which is not processed and full of additives). Obviously those of you who are into cooking will be fond of using salt to enhance flavours, but if your PMS symptoms are very bad, you really need to find other ways of sharpening the taste of your food – experiment with spices, herbs (sage is good), vinegars, lemon juice and nutritional yeast, which you can get in health-food shops. Try to do without table salt – again, try lemon juice or a dash of vinegar instead.

Exercise: Aim to exercise at least three times per week for one hour each time – or more often if you feel you have the energy. Walking, swimming, running or weights are all great ways to get fit and healthy, improve circulation and reduce your PMS effects. Basically, any form of exercise that you enjoy will be perfect!

Eat regularly: Eat small meals at regular intervals, leaving no more than three hours between meals. Choose plenty of whole-grain carbohydrates (e.g. brown bread, pasta or rice, whole-grain crackers) to maintain adequate blood sugar levels and prevent cells from being depleted of sugar and refilled with water. Avoid sugar as much as possible. Eat a diet high in colour. Fruit and vegetables that are full of colour are high in antioxidants and fantastic for your body.

Drink: Drink plenty of fluids, but not sugary drinks. Aim to drink a minimum of 2 litres of water a day and reduce your tea/coffee intake, although herbal teas can certainly help.

These simple changes will make such a difference to your fluid retention, not to mention your health. Give them a go for a month – I promise that you will see an improvement in your symptoms.

These simple changes will make such a difference to your fluid retention, not to mention your health.

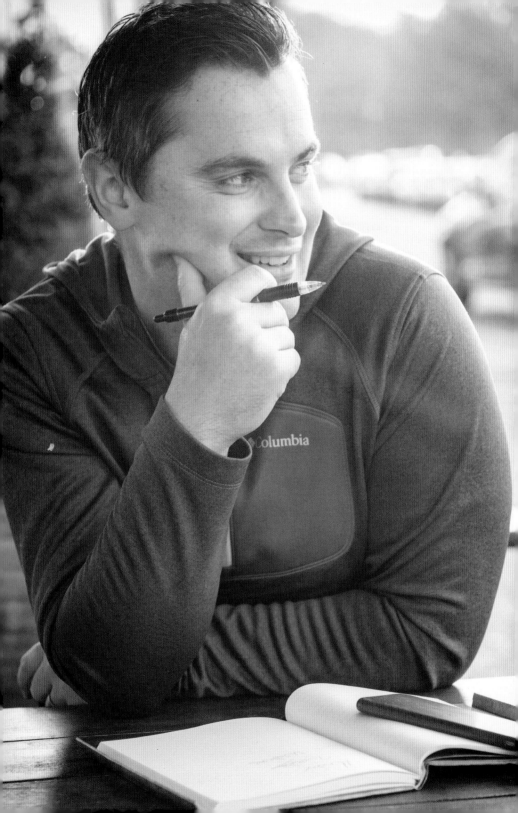

Wellbeing

One of the greatest benefits to improving your diet and fitness is getting a boost to your happiness levels.

22 MAKING THE BEST USE OF YOUR TIME

When it comes to getting healthy, assessing your time is a surprisingly crucial factor. Just like using a food diary to track what you're eating, or taking measurements of your body and the state it's in, seeing how you're spending your time can be equally valuable.

Did you know that…

- 39 per cent of Irish people sit for 5 to 10 hours each day?
- 31 per cent of people across the world sit for over 10 hours each day?
- on average, we spend 94 to 110 minutes per day commuting?
- Irish people aged 15-plus watched TV for an average of three hours and six minutes each day in July 2016*?

Let's do the maths. There are 168 hours in the week. If you get an average of eight hours' sleep a night – and for the sake of this exercise, let's assume you are getting a proper amount of sleep – that leaves 112 hours in the week to spend your time between work and play.

Keeping this in mind, I want you to fill out Table 1. This table breaks down how you are currently spending your time. Each box represents a different aspect of your week. Basically, anywhere you spend a

* Department of Health's Healthy Ireland Survey 2016

quantity of your time gets a box. Jot down how many hours you spend in each box every week. The total hours should add up to no more than 112.

Table 1: Your current week

WORK:	FAMILY:	FRIENDS:
COMMUTING:	TV:	SHOPPING:
EATING OUT:	PARTNER:	TIME FOR SELF:

This simple exercise will show you pretty quickly how you are spending your time. More often than not, people are surprised at their time spread, and particularly at the amount of time spent watching TV. It's kind of scary when you write it down!

Now I want you to do the exercise again, using the same categories. This time, I want you to fill out what you would change if you could to make your life healthier. Where would you spend more or less time? What would you adapt? Spend a few minutes doing this, and again the total should be no more than 112.

I realize that some things can't be changed – work is the obvious one. But don't forget that changes don't have to be massive to give you more time – for instance, you might realize that with a bit of planning, you could halve the time you spend doing your grocery shop.

Table 2: Your healthier week

WORK:	FAMILY:	FRIENDS:
COMMUTING:	TV:	SHOPPING:
EATING OUT:	PARTNER:	TIME FOR SELF:

This is going to be a timetable for the healthier you. Jot down a copy and put it somewhere you will see it regularly. It is a goal to work towards. By making a conscious decision to watch less TV, in particular, you will find that you have time to do things that make you healthier.

TURN RED ZONES INTO GREEN ZONES

Finding more hours in your week to focus on your diet and fitness goals is great, but don't write off all the other hours. The ways that you spend the hours in your day need to be tailored towards health in every way possible. From your car to your desk to your kitchen, you need to turn these from unhealthy to healthy zones – from red to green.

Not organizing yourself for your day will slowly sabotage all your efforts.

Not organizing yourself for your day will slowly sabotage all your efforts. Remember the old saying, 'If you fail to plan, you are planning to fail'? Well, nowhere is it more apt than when it comes to getting healthier.

So, take a look at your day from start to finish. Most people's lives fall into these zones: morning, travel to work, work/lunch/work, travel from work, home, weekends. Of course, there will be lots of variety depending on your circumstances, but you get the general idea – it's all about engineering things so that the healthier option is always available! Here are some simple tips to make each zone healthier:

Morning
- Don't rush straight into the shower – do a few gentle stretches first.
- Before your shower, have a glass of warm water and lemon.
- If you want to get in a run, walk or workout session in the morning, leave your gear out the night before.

- Prepare your breakfast the night before – try my Super-simple Overnight Oats (page 76).

Commuting to and from work
- Have some healthy snacks in your bag in case you missed breakfast or you are hungry at the end of the day.
- Get off the bus or train one stop earlier.
- Read something positive.
- Use the time for planning – put together a goal list.
- If you're driving, check your posture and keep checking it – make sure your head is erect, your shoulders relaxed and your tummy pulled in.
- Keep a bottle of water in your car.
- Download a motivational podcast to listen to. Alternatively, try to work on your stress levels by listening to your favourite music or comedy show.

Office
- Use the stairs – great for your lungs, your legs and also your stress levels. It gets easier in time!
- On a Monday, stock up with fruit and nuts for healthy snacking during your mid-morning and mid-afternoon breaks throughout the week. But try not to graze continually.
- Keep a large bottle or jug of water on your desk and make sure you finish it by the end of the day.
- Keep herbal teabags at your desk if they are not provided and try to alternate tea and coffee with herbal tea.
- Walk around to colleagues' desks instead of emailing about everything.
- Stand more.
- Switch to a Swiss ball instead of an office chair – see if you can get a standing desk.
- If you're arranging meetings, avoid putting out plates of pastries and biscuits – most people don't need them! If you need to provide snacks, make them healthy snacks.
- Can you have standing or walking meetings?

Identify like-minded colleagues who would be open to this.

Lunch
- Bring in a healthy lunch – you'll save money and calories!
- If you can't bring in a packed lunch, take a walk to buy it.
- Aim to make your lunch mainly protein with vegetables.
- Switch off your phone for 30 minutes.
- Take a walk. If you can't go outside because of the weather, or some other reason, try to walk around the building, and if there are stairs, go up and down them a few times.

Time at home
- Have your workout gear ready for when you get home – leave your running shoes by the front door.
- Get your workout session done before you sit down.
- Have your kitchen stocked with healthy foods.
- Know what you're going to have for dinner, ideally protein and vegetables.
- Don't have caffeine after 7 p.m.
- If they will last, put leftovers from dinner into a container for lunch at the office the following day.
- Prepare your breakfast.
- Get your gear sorted for the morning if you're planning to exercise.
- Don't look at any screens in your bedroom!

Weekends
- Time for planning, food shopping and meal prepping for the week!
- Try to carve out some time for proper relaxation.
- If you are going out for dinner, check if the restaurant has its current menus online – read them at home after you've eaten (so you're not hungry and easily tempted) and identify

the healthiest options. When you get to the restaurant, you can make your choices quickly and put the menu aside. Instead, focus your attention on the company and the conversation.

- Before you go out, have a small snack – say, a dozen almonds – to take the edge off your hunger so you avoid eating a lot of bread and nibbles before the meal.
- Keep in mind all the tips for handling alcohol at the end of Chapter 7 (page 54).

23 GETTING A GOOD NIGHT'S SLEEP

If you sleep for eight hours a night, that's 56 hours of your week spent sleeping. And if you sleep seven hours a night – and most experts recommend at least seven hours' sleep – that's 49 hours. Recently, I heard the Irish rugby star Gordon Darcy giving a talk and he gets ten hours of quality sleep every night to keep himself in the best possible condition. While we are not all professional athletes, hearing that makes you realize just how important sleep is.

Sleep is one of the key parts of your day. There is nothing that won't improve if you improve your sleep, and it is a key factor in losing weight. Good-quality sleep gives your mind a rest and a chance to process the events of the day. It gives your digestive system a breather and your hormones time to level out so that they do the work they are meant to do in regulating your appetite and managing your blood sugars. And it gives your muscles time to recover from exercise.

Here are some simple tips that will really improve the quality of your sleep:

GET A GOOD MATTRESS

You spend about one-third of your year – over 120 days – on your mattress, yet very few people actually invest in a good one. What may seem expensive in the short term will save you money in the long term.

A good mattress will help you sleep better, reduce back and joint pain and give you more energy.

Different types of mattresses will suit different people, so take your time in choosing yours. Personally, I have a King Koil mattress and I find it makes a big difference to my back and my sleep patterns too. I bought one after sleeping so well in a hotel that I had to find out the make and model of their mattress. I have never looked back!

CHANGE YOUR PILLOWS

The second most important thing after your mattress is your pillows. If you wake up with pain in your neck, either side of your neck or your upper back, much of this can be linked to your pillows. Trial and error is the best method here. Personally, I love memory-foam pillows, which mould to your sleeping position, but different pillows work for different people. Again, you will be amazed at how much of a difference it makes to your sleep.

INVEST IN BLACKOUT BLINDS

Our ancestors could teach us a lot about sleeping. Often older buildings include interior window shutters that, when closed, make bedrooms completely dark at night. If you've ever stayed in a country-house hotel with window shutters, you will know how well you can sleep there. Darkness improves the depth of our sleep, yet most of our bedrooms have lots of light seeping in, meaning that you never really get the deep sleep that your body needs. Invest in a set of blackout blinds and see the difference it makes to your sleep. You will fall asleep quicker and more deeply with no light in the room. Try to obscure any standby lights too – it's amazing how much light a tiny little standby light gives off in

There is nothing that won't improve if you improve your sleep...

a dark room. (Of course, ideally you won't have any technology in your bedroom in the first place!)

AVOID CAFFEINE AND REDUCE SUGAR AFTER SEVEN

Caffeine is a stimulant that can provide a great kick-start to your day and improve concentration all day. No doubt about it. But taken later in the afternoon and especially in the evening, it can stop you from getting a good night's sleep. Coffee, tea and green tea are all sources of caffeine and caffeine keeps you alert, which is the opposite of what you want to do when you sleep. So later in the day, switch to a peppermint, camomile or another herbal tea to relax the body and help you to unwind.

The same goes for reducing your sugar intake. Sugar will cause your energy levels to spike, so aim to avoid any sugars late at night.

For obvious reasons, having a big meal late at night and revving up your digestive system is not good for sleep. If you know you won't get to eat until late, you're better off eating a big lunch and making your late meal something lighter and protein-based. If your only opportunity to eat is late at night, try to go for things that will fill you up without taxing the digestive system too much – a bowl of soup and some wholemeal bread, a chicken sandwich, again made with wholemeal bread.

GO TECH-FREE BEFORE SLEEP

Technology – from televisions to iPads to game consoles – all stimulate the mind and can stop you from sleeping soundly. Stay away from these for at least 30 minutes before you go to sleep.

This is especially true if you have a TV in your bedroom. If you do one thing and one thing only to improve your sleep, it is to remove the TV from your bedroom. Instead, use those last 30 minutes to read a book or a magazine. Reading instead of viewing will help to improve your sleep no end!

KEEP A NOTEBOOK AND PEN BESIDE YOUR BED

If you struggle to get to sleep, or wake up a lot during the night, then one of the easiest ways around this is to have a notepad and pen beside your bed. Before you go to bed, make a list of all the things you didn't get to today that you want to get done tomorrow. Whatever is in your mind, just get it out of your head and written down. If you wake up during the night thinking about stuff, again, write it down. Writing things down really helps your mind to settle.

Reading instead of viewing will help to improve your sleep no end!

24 THE IMPORTANCE OF POSITIVE THINKING

If you sometimes find life a bit of a trudge and struggle to maintain your mood, working on your diet and fitness can really help. I am not a psychologist and I don't claim to be any kind of happiness expert, but from my experience with clients, I know that one of the greatest benefits to improving your diet and fitness is getting a boost to your happiness levels. Having more energy, feeling better and looking fitter has a powerful effect, making you feel motivated, confident and happy. And all the self-help/positive-thinking/motivational/ inspirational books in the world won't make any difference if you are really unfit and eating a lot of high-GI processed foods.

Think about the people you know who are consistently happy – and by that I don't mean the life and soul of the party. What I mean is people who approach most days positively. Those who seem to be able to handle stress and juggle the demands on them calmly and with good humour most of the time. Who are reasonable and considerate in how they deal with family, colleagues, friends. And who have reserves in the tank to cope with the occasional curve ball that life throws at them. Obviously there are personality factors at play in all of this. Mother Nature made some of us naturally more positive and resilient than others. But chances are the people who come to mind – who are in consistently good form, living a balanced life and handling stress well – also look healthy and fit.

It sounds like a dramatic statement, but sugar is one of the greatest everyday barriers to happiness. Eating to cope with stress or upset or sadness is a vicious circle. It might be that there are no easy or quick ways of resolving whatever is upsetting you, whereas food is available and you know it'll be a distraction and make you feel better. Chances are you reach for high-GI foods that will give you an initial lift, but when your blood sugars crash, you'll feel low and crave another 'fix'. And so you eat more foods that are high in calories, high in sugar and preservatives and bad for your health. It's a bit of a merry-go-round that is hard to get off. Stabilize your blood sugar levels by eating more healthily and you'll avoid those highs and lows and feel better.

It is not an extreme claim to say that in many cases, both depression and mood-related disorders can be helped with healthy eating and exercise. Both the experts and people who struggle with depression themselves all advocate a good diet and exercise as being very helpful for improving mental health. When you think of it, avoiding sugar crashes that sap your energy, and getting an endorphin boost from exerting yourself, are going to be good for your mind as well as your body.

Having asked you to measure everything else, I now want you to measure your happiness. The table overleaf is very simple. At the end of each day, I want you to rate how happy you feel on a scale of one to ten, one being extremely negative and ten being extremely positive.

Be honest. Put down a number that truly relates to how you feel, to how your day really was (copy the chart into a notebook if you're concerned about

It is not an extreme claim to say that in many cases both depression and mood-related disorders can be helped with healthy eating and exercise.

anyone else seeing it). The idea is that as you start to get healthy – eating better and exercising more – you will begin to see your mood improve.

	MON	TUES	WED	THURS	FRI	SAT	SUN	TOTAL
WK 1								
WK 2								
WK 3								
WK 4								

By using this chart to record how you feel, you will be able to see the direct relationship between what you eat, how much you move and how you feel. And by eating real foods and exercising more, things will change.

What type of person are you? A glass-half-full or half-empty type? Do you always see the negatives in a situation or the positives? It is no surprise that this is one of the key aspects of real happiness. Most people probably fall somewhere in the middle – both sensibly optimistic (hopeful but not 'on a high' the whole time) and sensibly pessimistic (cautious but open to new people and experiences).

If you are habitually negative, or notice yourself becoming more pessimistic, this can be detrimental to your wellbeing because how you see situations shapes your thoughts, and your thoughts can dictate your mood. In other words, you don't have gloomy and negative thoughts because you're in a low mood; rather, you're in a low mood because your thoughts are negative.

What this means is that while it sometimes seems as though moods are like the weather – something that comes over us and can't be controlled – we can actually do a lot to manage our thinking and therefore our moods.

Successful and contented people tend to be positive in their outlook when it comes to work, partners, family, friendships, community – everything. Being positive helps to…

- lower resting heart rate
- improve digestion
- improve sleep quality
- lower stress levels
- reduce visceral fat storage
- reduce weight
- reduce your chances of getting sick
- make you feel more fulfilled

To improve your level of positivity, start by analysing your life as it is now. What is causing you to be negative? And what are the barriers to feeling more positive? Don't edit yourself – just make a list of the top five things you believe are making you feel negative.

Now that you have made your list, I want you to look at each one and think what you could change about it. Some things might be relatively straightforward. For instance, if your house is a mess and it's getting you down, could you plan to declutter and reorganize, one room at a time, over the next month or two? Can you identify a regular weekly time to do that? Maybe get a friend on board? Or could you make it a family project for the next few months?

Or if you're feeling bad about having lost touch with an old friend, could you clear an hour to draft a nice message that you can send by email or card to express how sorry you are that you haven't been in touch and saying that you'd love to meet for a coffee next time they're free?

Successful and contented people tend to be positive in their outlook when it comes to work, partners, family, friendships, community - everything.

If you are dealing with challenges such as illness, bereavement, unemployment or disability, of course I don't want to suggest that there is an easy solution. But if you can break down your situation and look at your daily routine, is there any support you can get for any part of it that will ease the pressure? Either informally – through your network of family and friends – or formally via agencies and support groups?

If you do this exercise regularly, breaking down the negatives in your life and looking at practical ways of addressing them, it will become a really useful tool in helping you to become more positive in your outlook.

MANAGING THE SEASONAL CHANGES IN YOUR HAPPINESS

25

For many people, the changing of the seasons seems to have a big impact on happiness and health. Mood and energy levels are hugely affected by the time of year, and this in turn affects weight and general health. Seasonal Affective Disorder (SAD) can arise in any season of the year, but for most people who are affected, the lack of light in winter is the trigger. Symptoms of SAD include the following:

- Difficulty waking up in the morning.
- Tendency to oversleep.
- Lack of energy.
- Tendency to overeat and especially a craving for carbohydrates.
- Weight gain.
- Negative outlook on life.
- Decreased sex drive.
- Withdrawal from friends, family and social activities.

If you find that you suffer from these symptoms at the same time of year every year, you may suffer from SAD. It can have a big impact on your life and your health so it's encouraging to realize that there is a lot you can do to diminish its effects.

EXERCISE

Exercise is possibly the most important tool to help with any form of mood disorder, no matter what that disorder is. When you exercise at any effort level, you are taking time away from the stresses of life, getting your blood pumping and releasing some endorphins into your system. As you know, endorphins are the hormones that make you feel good. They will change your outlook on your day, your week and your month.

But to get the most from your exercise, you need to ensure that you are exercising hard enough. Every session you do, you have to hit the 'talk test' point (page 160), ensuring that you are slightly out of breath, but still able to talk.

COPY THE OPTIMISTS!

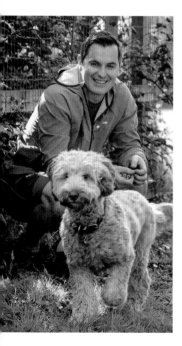

Optimists are always glass-half-full people, no matter what happens. If you're not a natural optimist, it can feel a bit strange to fake it. But try. Use the positive-thinking exercise I recommended earlier. And you don't have to 'put on' a mood. It's a question of taking practical steps to copy what optimists do naturally. For instance, Irish people generally love to moan and give out about other people. That's fine when it's just letting off steam, but if you're constantly down on everything, you're bringing yourself down as well. Try to see the good in people and situations. Don't assume the worst of people.

Whatever your outlook on life – positive or negative – chances are that you will surround yourself with people who are similar. As a good friend and colleague of mine, Neil O'Brien, says, 'Twos attract twos and tens attract tens!' So, on a scale of one to ten, are you a two or a ten? However you rate yourself may be keeping you in a bubble of positivity or negativity. The more negativity you surround yourself with the unhappier you will be. Embrace your positive friends and be careful about how you're influenced by people who bring out your negative side.

GET SOME LIGHT

If you are affected by SAD in winter, why not book a few days away when the days are short? Not only does this ensure that you get more light, and heat too if you book somewhere warm, it also gives you something to look forward to. It gives you a reason to get out of bed, to work productively and to be healthy. It may seem like a simple thing but it is surprisingly effective.

Another strategy for dealing with the winter lack of light is getting a SAD light. These are not cheap but if getting the winter blues is an annual problem for you, investing in one of these is worth considering. They transmit white or blue light that triggers an increase in serotonin, an important brain chemical that helps with everything from mood, to sleep, to appetite, but which runs down in the darker winter months. You will find information on SAD lights online.

Getting more colour into your life is possibly the simplest recommendation of all.

BRIGHTEN UP YOUR LIFE

Getting more colour into your life is possibly the simplest recommendation of all. Surround yourself with dark colours all the time and you will find that this has a direct impact on your mood and on your day. Optimistic, happy, positive people generally wear colour, not all black or monochrome. Try to surround yourself with bright, vibrant colours and see what a difference they make to how you feel and to your outlook on life.

26 PLANNING FOR HAPPINESS

When you are happier, you come across as more confident, capable, open and friendly, and that creates opportunities – in work, in your personal life, in your social and community life. And when it comes to the challenges – well, I have used the term 'the virtuous circle' before, and that's what happens when you begin to feel more in control of your life. You become more committed to looking after yourself and to following good eating and exercise routines. You sleep better and you have more energy for what life throws at you. And, in turn, the challenges end up being less daunting and more manageable. Here are some more tips for working on your happiness:

START SMALL

By making changes that are too big, you can set yourself up for failure. From all the content in this book, pick just one thing you can do this week – one thing that seems incredibly easy, that you know won't mean you have to make too many changes to your week. Next week, pick another thing and add it in.

SET GOALS AND MAKE PLANS

It gives a sense of purpose and is incredibly rewarding to set targets and then hit them. So when you're ready, I encourage you to use the material in this book to clarify what's important to you and set short-, medium- and long-term goals around your health and wellbeing. But don't set too many of them at once. Set a few to be going on with and put in a review date.

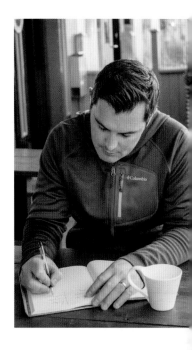

- Once you've set your goals, visualize what it will be like to achieve them.
- Plan to do one thing every day to help you achieve your goals.
- In order to do that, try to get better at planning – make lists of what you need to get done each day.

On your to-do list every few days – at least once a week – include something new or something that scares you. You'll get a huge boost from doing something you've never tried before or didn't think you could do.

PLAN A TREAT

Identify what your treat is going to be in a few weeks' time. You are making big changes to your life, so give yourself a tangible reward to work towards: clothes, books, holidays – anything that you love – are all great rewards that you can use. You will be far more motivated as a result and it's a great pattern to get into – setting a goal, planning a timeframe and following up with a reward.

FIND HAPPY PEOPLE

Your social network is one of the most important elements of health and it's simple to develop it. You may already know a group of people who go out and do healthy things together or share a common interest. Well, if you want to join them, pick up the phone or send a text. It is one of the first steps you can take that will have such a big impact on your happiness. If you don't already know of one, seek out a group in your area – there's bound to be one.

By making changes that are too big, you can set yourself up for failure.

At the same time, reduce your social-media time. It's better to go out and connect with real people than to stay glued to a phone or computer. And since a lot of social-media activity is about showing off, you're better off rationing your time on it.

BE KIND

Treat yourself kindly. If you fall off the wagon, don't beat yourself up.

Treat yourself kindly. If you fall off the wagon, don't beat yourself up. Take a look at why it happened – was your plan too hard, too stressful, too much too soon? Think ahead and do something else to make the changes. Don't give up. Just keep going until you find the tools that work for you. When you stop fighting change and find your perfect mix of planning and activities, you will feel a greater sense of ownership about your health and ultimately be happier.

Be kind to other people too. Smile more and give someone a compliment each day. Whatever you give out will come back to you with interest!

COUNT YOUR BLESSINGS

Take a look at just how far you have come, rather than looking at how far you have to go. We often have a vision of the person we 'should' be and we beat ourselves up for not being that person. But look what you have done and the differences that you have made already. Be proud of that. Realize that what you have in your life is fantastic. It's great to aim for more but important to recognize the value of what you have.

MOVE MORE AND EAT LESS SUGAR

I could not omit this from my top tips on how to be happier!

GET A PET!

I love animals. As I grow older, I love them more and more. No matter how hard, long or stressful my day is, all of that changes when I come in the door. I find coming home to a house with two cats and a dog is wonderfully de-stressing. Pets are great in helping to make you mindful – no matter what's going on, you can put it to one side and just focus on them. Indeed, even as I write this, my wife and I are about to welcome a second dog because we are so enamoured with our first!*

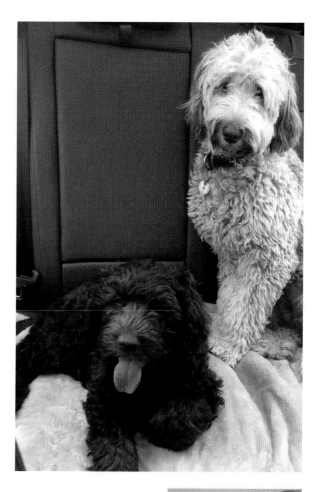

Pets are a commitment – some more than others – and it's important that when choosing a pet, you match them to your resources and the level of time and involvement you can give them. But if you can bring a pet into your life, you will get so much from them in terms of enjoyment, escapism, relaxation and love.

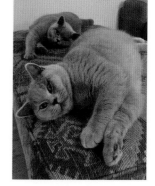

* Since completing the book Woody – left in the picture – arrived to join his half-sister Sophie. And the cats are brothers Hamish (front) and Harry.

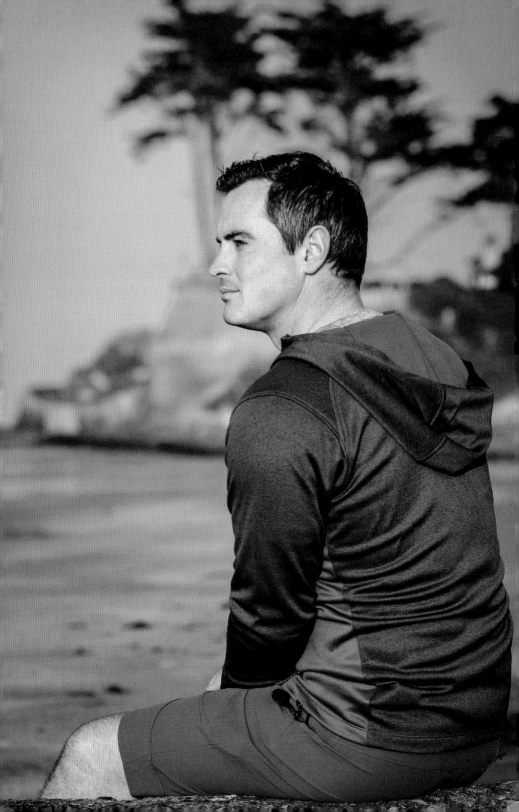

Simple but effective tips to help you stay on track

When the going gets tough, you will need to dig deep and push on through. At those times, remind yourself of what triggered your decision to change.

27 TOP TIPS FOR WEIGHT LOSS

1 EAT REGULAR MEALS

Eating meals throughout the day will help keep your metabolism stable as well as burning calories all day long. When we don't eat for an extended amount of time, it slows down the body, reducing the number of calories you naturally burn during the day. Don't skip breakfast. There is a great debate about whether it's best to eat three main meals or five smaller meals a day. I tend to go with three meals and two snacks, but see what suits you best. Your snacks can be fruit or small meals full of nutrients. No matter which way you choose to eat, keep your diet low in high-sugar and high-GI foods, just like in recipes I have in this book. These two factors are not only bad for your waistline; they are bad for your health.

2 EAT WHOLE FRESH FOODS

For foods to last a long time on our shelves, they have to be filled with preservatives. These deplete the nutrients and vitamins originally found in these foods. When possible, purchase fresh foods and avoid pre-packaged and convenient fast food, as these types of food are typically higher in calories, fat and salt as well as preservatives. If you have local markets in your area, then why not pick up your fruit and veg there? You will get fresher produce and you will be supporting the local economy too.

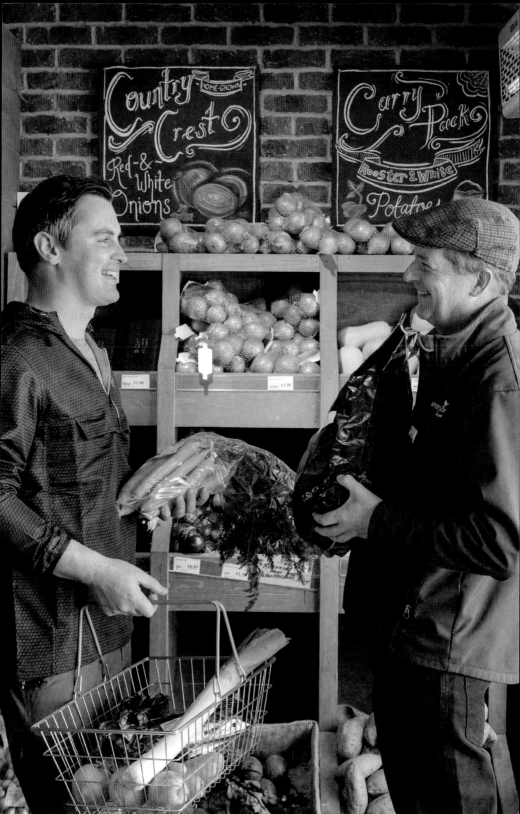

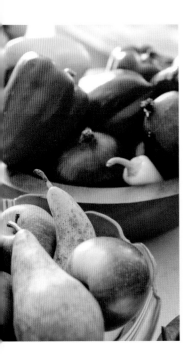

3 EAT A DIET FULL OF COLOUR

All of your meals should have plenty of colour – it's a handy way of ensuring that you are getting enough vegetables and fruit. Vegetables and fruit are packed with fibre, vitamins, minerals and antioxidants and are very low in calories. They help keep you satisfied longer, are a great snack and can be eaten with every meal. Most Irish people don't eat enough vegetables, but with such a great selection in our shops, there really is no excuse, so load up your plate!

4 EAT WHOLE GRAINS

Eat brown carbs, not white. This is one of the easiest ways to improve your diet. Whole grains are unrefined products that have maintained their nutritional and fibre content. An additional benefit of eating 100 per cent whole grains, such as breads and pastas, is that they help maintain blood sugar levels and keep you fuller for longer.

5 EAT THE RIGHT FATS

Fat has a reputation for being bad for us, but most fats are fine in moderation and indeed our body needs a certain amount of fat. The key thing to avoid is eating trans fats – these will lead to weight gain and increase your risk of cardiovascular disease.

6 BEWARE OF LIQUID CALORIES

Extra calories can add up quickly – for example, a 500ml can of fizzy drink can contain 10 teaspoons of sugar. These types of calories will not fill you up, nor provide any nutritional value, but they will pile on the pounds. Even the supposedly healthy soft drinks and juices contain huge quantities of sugar. Fizzy drinks or diet drinks have no place in a healthy diet, so switch to water instead. Be wise with your alcohol consumption. Alcohol is also full of empty calories, so make it an occasional treat.

7 BE A DETECTIVE WITH FOOD LABELS

When reading the list of ingredients on packaged foods, if you do not recognize the ingredient or cannot pronounce it, perhaps this isn't something you want to be putting in your body. If you see a product with a huge list of ingredients, put the item right back on the shelf. You really want to look at the sugar content – remember, 4g of sugar is the equivalent of 1 teaspoon. If it's high – more than 2 teaspoons per serving – put it back on the shelf.

8 TREAT YOURSELF

We all have those few foods that we know aren't good for us, yet we have a hard time avoiding them. The more you tell yourself you can't have them, the more you want them and the harder your health journey becomes. Eventually you will rebel and eat as much of that restricted food as you can. So allow yourself a treat from time to time, but remember to keep it within moderation. Make it a once-a-week treat – this way you aren't cutting the food from your diet. There is even evidence that if you give your body a treat just once a week, your metabolism speeds up to burn it off. So it's not only good for your mood and morale, but also for your body and your long-term health.

9 GIVE YOUR STOMACH TIME TO CATCH UP

It takes our bodies up to 20 minutes to realize we have had enough to eat. Because of this delay in

When reading the list of ingredients on packaged foods, if you do not recognize the ingredient or cannot pronounce it, perhaps this isn't something you want to be putting in your body.

feeling full, it is very easy to eat more than our bodies actually need, leaving us feeling overfull. Think of that stuffed feeling you get after Christmas dinner, where your body makes you sleepy because it needs all its energy to digest the food that you have put into it! You need to slow down your eating – put your knife and fork down between each bite – and chew your food thoroughly. Your stomach expands and shrinks in relation to the quantity of food you put into it and over time it becomes used to receiving large volumes. By slowing down your eating, you will eat less and your stomach will adapt and become used to receiving a smaller volume, meaning it will feel full with less food. It's another way in which our bodies can actually help us lose weight and keep it off.

10 GET MOVING

Your body was not meant to sit all day long. For overall health, and especially to strengthen all your muscles, including your heart, you need daily exercise. Exercise can also help you sleep better and improve your mood. So whether it's a high-impact workout at the gym or a walk at lunchtime, get moving! Ideally you should be doing a minimum of 30 minutes each day of vigorous exercise. The next chapter has my top tips to motivate you to get fit but in the meantime here are some tips to help you move more:

- Have you ever noticed how people compete to park as close as possible to the shops? **Park a little further away** and let your feet do the rest.

- An old one, but a goodie – **get off the bus or train one stop earlier** and walk a little further to work. As you get fitter, you can make it two stops, three stops, etc. It's a simple way to get a little bit more movement into your day.

- Standing is great for your body, so put it to work more – **stand at regular intervals during the day.**

- If you're at a desk all day, **take the recommended screen breaks.** You are supposed to do this anyway for your eyes and your back, and it's a great opportunity to move (can you walk downstairs and back up again, or to another part of the building and back?).

- **Carry your bags.** Carrying groceries and shopping bags in general is a simple way to get more weight-bearing exercise into your day.

- **Keep your house clean!** Household chores often involve a lot of movement and you may be more motivated to do them when you realize that you're also doing your body good.

28 TOP TIPS FOR FITNESS

1 MAKE MOVEMENT A PART OF YOUR DAY

Exercise is something that so many people consider an activity to be done several times a week, and this may be true, but I also firmly believe that you should get as much exercise (i.e. movement) into your day as possible. Apart from getting off the bus early or using stairs instead of lifts, which I've mentioned already, here's another simple thing you can do that has huge health benefits: stand more.

Stand any time you get the chance – on the bus or train into work, in waiting rooms, etc. The more you sit, the less your body has to do, so standing is far better for your back, your heart and just your overall wellbeing. Standing a little more during the day will help to increase energy expenditure, burning 50 to 70 calories an hour more than sitting. If you stand for four hours extra per day, that's an extra 200 to 280 calories a day, or around 2lbs of fat a month.

2 ENJOY YOURSELF!

Life is too short to spend it doing exercise you hate. And it's also too short not to exercise at all! So many people choose activities that they don't enjoy as they think it will help them lose weight or tone up, but inevitably it becomes tedious and they stop doing it. Try different exercises until you find something you enjoy. When you find an exercise you enjoy, you feel alive and excited and you are far more likely to stick with it. There is such a great choice out there; it is just a matter of trial and error.

3 DO TWO MINUTES A DAY

Everyone has at least two minutes a day! If you've never exercised or haven't for a long time and you feel very unfit and scared, then just pick two resistance exercises from the ones I have given you in Chapter 20 and do as many reps as you can in 60 seconds. Do this for seven days, ideally picking two different exercises every day, and you will be surprised at the difference it makes to how you feel and also to your mindset. The following week, you will be ready to do five minutes.

4 WALK OR RUN?

Both are fantastic and will deliver great results in terms of your cardiovascular and overall health – once you are working hard enough! It's very easy to go for a long walk but not move at a hard enough pace to bring fitness benefits. So do the 'talk test' (page 160) and if you're not slightly out of breath as you talk, increase your pace. Once you're working hard enough, it doesn't make that much difference which you do, so see point 2 here – do the one you enjoy the most because you will stick with it.

Life is too short to spend it doing exercise you hate.

5 TIMING

There is no ideal time to exercise for your body. You will get great benefits whether you train in the morning or evening. Again, it's all about doing what you enjoy most and will stick with in the long term. If you are a morning person, train in the morning. If you are an evening person, train in the evening.

6 GET A TRAINING BUDDY

If you find you are losing motivation, why don't you try to start a small exercise group with your friends, each person taking it in turns to organize the sessions and the logistics? Group support and working together to achieve a common goal can make such a big difference to how motivated you feel. I have a WhatsApp group with my own friends and we use it to push each other to do more races and train harder. Give it a try and you will find that you stay focused for longer.

7 REGISTER FOR AN EVENT

If you find you are losing motivation, why don't you try to start a small exercise group with your friends.

If you are target driven, then why not log on to www.runireland.com or www.activeeurope.com and register for an event? Print out your receipt and place it somewhere visible. Once you have registered, it's time to build your training plan and then just work towards the event, ticking the boxes each week as you get the sessions done. It's a great way to stay focused and driven and the best part of all is completing it and crossing the finish line. That becomes the addictive part (not to mention getting the medal and the T-shirt!)…

8 BOOK A SESSION WITH A PERSONAL TRAINER

If all else fails, jumpstart your training by booking a session with a personal trainer. During the session, discuss everything that holds you back and every question you have. Nail down some goals that you want to work towards and let the trainer use their experience and skills to help you get back on track in the right way. Maybe even book a follow-up session for two months later and use that as a target to aim for. Personal trainers are perfectly happy to see people on a one-off basis like this. We do it all the time.

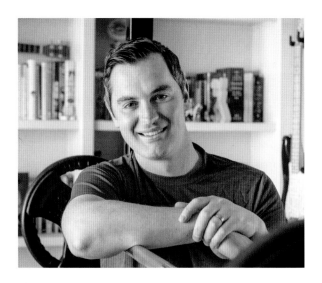

9 CHANGE IT UP

When you see results, you stay focused and driven,
and if you want to keep getting results from your
training, change it regularly. You can change the
speed, distance, weight, workout routine, class or
anything at all, really!

10 RECOVERY

Recovery is a key component of fitness, helping your
body to get results faster. Ideally aim to get some
nutrients into your body in the first 20 minutes after
each session. Protein-based foods such as eggs, fish
and meat are ideal for this, or if you're on the go, milk
or flavoured milk is a perfect recovery food too. If you
choose a protein shake, make it the one with the least
amount of added sugar!

29 TOP TIPS FOR FAMILY HEALTH

One of the most important aspects of both individual and national wellbeing is health in the family. If every family in Ireland improved its health, then we would be setting up the next generation for a far brighter future. Yet households all over Ireland are struggling with health issues due to a lack of knowledge and time, a sense of helplessness about how complicated healthier living is and where to start, and maybe an inability to work together to get healthy. I hope that the information between these covers will convince you that getting healthy is not complicated and that you can take it in simple steps, one at a time. Here are some tips for working as a family to improve everyone's health:

1 SET AN EXAMPLE

If you aren't prepared to improve your own health, then it's unfair to put pressure on others to do the same. Lecturing your children about health without leading by example won't work. The family unit has to get fit as a whole and parents need to lead by example. If you can do this, you will see a much better result.

2 SHOP SMART

Healthy living starts with what comes into the house. The food that goes into your trolley in the supermarket is crucial. You need to be firm that certain foods don't make it into your house – if it's not there your family can't eat it. Load up on all the foods I have in this book and you will be rocking!

- Read food labels and reduce your sugar and sodium intake.

- Change the colour of the foods that come into your house and go on to your plate. Aim for plenty of vegetables and fruit and lots of brown whole-grain carbohydrates.

- Eliminate drinks and cordials that contain sugar (including fruit juice) and instead go with water or water with fruit in it for flavour.

- Similarly, avoid sugary flavoured yoghurts. Instead, have Greek or natural yoghurt and add fruit and nuts to flavour it.

3 COOK

Education is so important when it comes to health, so why not ask each member of the house to cook one meal each week? They research the recipe, get the ingredients and cook the meal. Obviously if you have smaller children, either you, an older sibling or another adult will be doing most of the cooking, but they can still be involved every step of the way. Not only is it healthier, but it is also giving your children a tool for life. Freezing the leftovers is handy too, as you will have a freezer full of healthy dinners to eat. (Indeed, I love to batch cook and place the meals in the freezer so that during the week, I can eat healthily.)

4 EAT TOGETHER

Eat together at the table each day – a simple yet very effective tool not only for health, but also for

Lecturing your children about health without leading by example won't work. The family unit has to get fit as a whole ...

communication within the family. Research from the United States has shown that families who eat together have a far lower risk of obesity.

And remember, don't have a TV on in the background! And don't forget what I said about getting smaller plates. Swap your dinner plates for ones that are 10 per cent smaller and you'll be training your family to be satisfied by smaller portion sizes.

5 TREAT YOURSELVES

Don't be afraid to have a treat meal every now and again. By totally banishing takeaways, you will create a bad relationship with these foods. Instead, have them sporadically. However, try to avoid making a big deal out of the fact that you are 'breaking out' to eat foods your family normally doesn't eat. That just puts a high premium on them. Instead, make it a bit of fun and stress the social aspect as well.

6 CHANGE YOUR CHILDREN'S THINKING ABOUT TREATS

Having a 'treat' drawer or cupboard in your house makes it sound like these foods are both bad and exciting ... it makes these foods very tempting.

Following on from the previous point, get rid of the 'treat' drawer or cupboard. Traditionally, it is the drawer or cupboard that is full of crisps, biscuits, cakes and so on. I have used the idea of treat meals throughout the book, as it's a handy shorthand term. But having a 'treat' drawer or cupboard in your house makes it sound like these foods are both bad and exciting – the things everyone really wants to have instead of being forced to eat all the 'boring' healthy stuff! Either way, it makes these foods very tempting.

Of course, sweet and high-GI stuff is very attractive to us – I can't deny that – but we need to train ourselves and our children how to handle it. And one of the ways of doing that is to stop treating these foods as if they're the only ones that will really make us feel good, or as if they're the ultimate reward for good behaviour. Instead of having a treat drawer, involve your children in planning your family's treat meals as a routine part of your life and get them to invent healthy snacks (if you have time, they could help make some of the snack recipes in this book).

7 MOVE MORE

Have a car-free day once a week or make sure you only use the car for trips longer than a certain distance. This increases the amount of walking you do as a family.

Get some good rain-proof gear so your family doesn't see rain as an obstacle to going outdoors. While we may get a lot of rain, we live in a temperate climate and there is very little reason not to get outside most days if you're wearing the right gear.

If your lifestyle permits it, get a dog. There's nothing like having to walk a dog at least once a day to force you outdoors no matter what the weather. Dogs want to be walked 365 days a year! (Of course, if your children do what children often do and leave the parents walking the dog most of the time, that's OK – at least someone in the family is getting out the door.)

Have a car-free day once a week or make sure you only use the car for trips longer than a certain distance.

8 ACTIVITY-OF-CHOICE DAY

Every weekend or month, pick one day where a family member gets to choose an activity for the whole family. Ireland is awash with so many great sports; it offers so many opportunities to try different things. It will be a really enjoyable way of getting fitter together, and it's a chance for both you and your kids to sample different activities and perhaps find something new to add to your regular fitness routine.

9 DO YOUR CHORES!

Every bit of physical activity adds up and you'd be surprised at the range of movement involved in doing housework over one day. Share the workload so everyone can benefit.

10 SET FAMILY TARGETS

Focus on activity and making your kids feel good about what their bodies can do.

Get together as a family and set fitness and activity targets and put rewards in place for when you achieve them. Check in each week and work together to make sure you hit those targets. Make it all about health and fitness rather than weight loss to avoid the kids getting fixated on weight – yours or theirs. There is enough pressure on children already from social media and peers. If your children are overweight and you are gradually improving things using the information in this book, then unless there is an underlying medical issue, their weight will adjust to a healthy level. Avoid focusing on their size and instead focus on activity and making them feel good about the things their body can do.

TOP TIPS FOR A HEALTHY HOLIDAY 30

Holidays are fantastic and very beneficial to our health and wellbeing. Whether it's a staycation in Ireland, a city break, a beach holiday in Europe or something more adventurous, going on holiday is an opportunity to take time away from the usual routine, spend quality time with family or friends, explore new places or activities, and generally recharge.

Of course, holidays can also be challenging for your food and fitness plans – but only if you let them! If your mentality is that holidays are 'time off for good behaviour' or that somehow foreign calories don't count, or that you have no control over what happens on holiday, well, then you will undo some of your good work. On the other hand, if you approach it by saying that you are going to have a great time, enjoying everything your holiday destination has to offer, while still keeping up your good habits, then you have no reason to fear what will happen on holiday.

1 WEIGH YOURSELF BEFORE YOU GO

Knowing your weight before you travel and knowing that you will be checking it again when you come home is a good way to keep you focused when you're away and is likely to motivate you to do more exercise and to think twice before going up to the buffet for second helpings!

2 BE DEFINITE AT THE BUFFET

Unlimited food and drink encourages you to try everything on display and eat far more than you routinely would.

Buffet meals are a disaster when it comes to waistlines. Remember what I said earlier about portion and plate size and how optics affect the volume of food we consume? Well, unlimited food and drink encourages you to try everything on display and eat far more than you routinely would. For instance, if you normally eat cereal or eggs or fruit and yoghurt in the mornings, a breakfast buffet in a hotel will somehow give you the idea that you should have all three, and maybe a glass of juice and a bit of toast too – it would be a pity not to when everything looks so delicious and you're paying for it. After all, it's not often you get to relax over breakfast and it'll keep you going for the day (you tell yourself). And that's just breakfast.

Try to stick to one filling choice for breakfast, and for lunch and dinner stick to three actual courses – a salad, then protein and vegetables, and then a treat for dessert. One of each. Simple and effective. You may feel like you are getting the best value by indulging more, but stick to your structure and your waistline will thank you for it.

Of course, one way of avoiding the temptation of the buffet, as well as keeping closer tabs on what you're eating and your budget, is to go for self-catering accommodation. That way you can plan your meals and snacks for most of the day, enjoying the business of checking out the local markets and food shops, and then go out to dinner knowing that you've been eating wisely all day.

3 STOCK UP ON WATER

It can be so easy to order cocktails by the pool, not because you want them but because it's warm and you're thirsty. Instead, try to stock up on water when you arrive – buy a six-pack of 1.5-litre bottles of water – and have one beside you at all times during the day.

The same thing applies to ice creams and hot dogs and other things that call out to you during the day when you're on holiday. As often as not, you eat because you're thirsty rather than hungry.

4 GET YOUR EXERCISE DONE EARLY

There's no reason not to continue with your cardio and resistance training and stretching when you're on holiday. And the earlier you train, the more likely it is that you will do your session rather than find an excuse to skip it. The endorphins that will kick in will make you feel good and help you to stay motivated as well, and you're less likely to go overboard with food and drink later. So it's win-win all round.

5 ALCOHOL AT ONE MEAL ONLY

It can be all too easy to slip into the habit of having an aperitif before lunch, then alcohol at lunch, then a couple of drinks in the afternoon, and then more alcohol with dinner and finally a night-cap. Over the course of a day, you could easily consume the equivalent of a bottle, or even two bottles, of wine. (And I'm being conservative with that estimate!)

While alcohol has its place in helping you relax, hopefully you are already relaxed by being on holiday. Drinking throughout the day on holiday can simply be a habit ...

While alcohol has its place in helping you relax, hopefully you are already relaxed by being on holiday. Drinking through the day on holiday can simply be a habit, and it's one you can break if you focus on it. If you remember that alcohol is just liquid calories, it should help you keep it in its place. Being on holiday shouldn't be an excuse to go crazy. So enjoy a few drinks, but try to keep alcohol to just one meal. If you're thirsty, drink water.

6 USE YOUR FEET

If you have to go somewhere, then why not walk as opposed to getting a cab or bus? You're on holiday and not in any rush, the weather is good, so why not? The exercise will do your body the world of good and it's adding to your daily movement. Use the stairs to get around the hotel as opposed to using the lifts all the time.

7 KEEP A FOOD DIARY

Food diaries are a simple, cheap and surprisingly effective way of staying healthy. When you begin to write it down, you will be surprised at what you are actually consuming every day. My clients usually find it quite a wake-up call! It's a tool you can use at home, of course, but it's super-useful for keeping tabs on what you're eating on holiday.

8 GET YOUR FAMILY INVOLVED

Activities that the family can do together – walking, hiking, running, swimming, cycling, tennis – are a perfect way of exercising on holiday. There are lots of activities that are promoted for their fun or adventure aspects, which also involve a lot of physical movement. They are ideal for getting everyone moving and may even be your opportunity to get the family thinking about what activity you can all do together when you get home.

9 USE THE TIME TO PLAN

I always use my holidays to reflect on my current training and to look to the future. Taking the time to examine what I have done well and not so well, and learning from any mistakes that I have made along the way, is really helpful. Holidays are a good time to reflect on where you are and where you want to be and to map out what is going to be different when you get home.

10 ABOVE ALL, HAVE FUN AND DE-STRESS!

Stress is bad for your health, in lots of different ways. So above all, when on holiday, do whatever you can to relax and unwind and bring your stress levels down as much as possible.

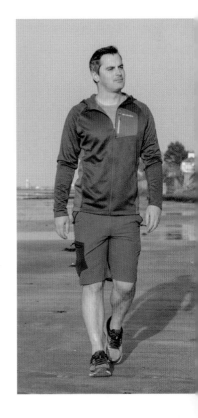

31 TOP TIPS FOR MANAGING STRESS

Life is tough, and there will be times when it throws something at you that will really challenge you and when getting through every day is a challenge. So here are some tips from my experience that will help you get through this.

1 TALK ABOUT IT

Stress can affect your mood, especially when you hold it in. Simply talking about how you are feeling can make a big difference. Men are especially bad at doing this, yet it can make such a difference to how you feel and how you handle pressure.

2 YOU WILL ALWAYS FEEL BETTER AFTER EXERCISE

Even when it is the very last thing you feel like doing, even if it's just a short burst, movement – intense movement, ideally – will make you feel better and help you manage your stress levels better. Endorphins are one of most effective natural lifts you can get.

3 KEEP EATING REAL FOOD

It's often so much easier to rely on convenience foods when you are busy and stressed, but these foods won't supply you with the nutrients you need. As much as you can, eat real food that you cook yourself. It is far healthier and better for you. No matter what time you eat or what you are eating, aim to get as much colour onto your plate as you can. Foods with colour are full of antioxidants and anti-inflammatory nutrients that will help your body to manage the effects of stress better.

4 DON'T BEAT YOURSELF UP

Sometimes in life things get in the way of your food and fitness plans. If you beat yourself up over it, it will only stress you out even more. Just accept that you can only do your best and that you will be able to get back on track when the time is right for you.

5 SET SMALLER GOALS

Big goals are great but if you're stuck for time it's going to be harder to hit them, so why not break them down into smaller, more achievable ones that you can do? No matter what your goal is, there are always ways to break it down into more manageable tasks. And hitting your goals every week will increase your motivation.

Just accept that you can only do your best and that you will be able to get back on track when the time is right for you.

6 WRITE IT DOWN AND MAP IT OUT

We all work better when we have plans in place. No matter what your problem is, you will feel better when it's mapped out in front of you. Get a blank page and get writing, organizing everything into a plan. Keep that plan handy and put a line through each step as you achieve it. You will be amazed at how much better you feel!

7 READ TO GET BETTER SLEEP

Books are a great way to help you sleep better. As I said in the chapter on sleep, you should stop looking at any screens at least 30 minutes before you want to go to sleep. Reading can provide an easy way to wean yourself off phones and TV screens before bed. By relaxing the mind before you go to sleep, you will improve the quality of the sleep that you actually get, leaving you feeling rested and relaxed when you wake up the next day. A nice, easy novel or some non-fiction about a topic that interests you is probably a better choice than a page-turning thriller!

8 KEEP MEASURING

I am a firm believer that we have to measure some health markers to stay healthy for life. Even when you're stressed, it's so important to keep measuring. Consistency is key no matter what, so don't let it slip. Structure is a great way to keep on pushing through the most stressful of times.

9 KEEP YOUR EYES ON THE PRIZE

No matter how stressed you get, just keep your goal in mind and work towards it. Have a reward in place for when you hit it so that you can enjoy the moment when it's done.

10 DO THIS RELAXATION TECHNIQUE

Relaxation is about switching off from your day and focusing on your breathing and your body, rather than what's going on in your head. This is a method I have used for a long time, especially before any lectures or TV work, when my stress levels are through the roof. It is one of the best techniques that I have come across to provide pretty much instant relaxation and it can be used anywhere, even while working at your desk.

- Start by closing your eyes, focusing on your breathing. Breathe in through your nose and out through your mouth. Ensure that you are drawing air into the pit of your stomach on the inhalation and emptying your lungs fully on the exhalation.

- Now breathe in for around five seconds and out for about five seconds. That's one set. Repeat for five to ten sets, depending on how much time you have.

- Next, breathe in for five seconds. Then hold your breath for five seconds while tensing your calf muscles. Breathe out for five seconds as you relax your calf muscles. That's one set. Repeat for three sets.

- Now use the same technique on each of the following, for three sets each:

  - Quads
  - Fists
  - Forearms
  - Arms
  - Shoulders
  - Back

- Finally, it's time to apply the technique to the whole body. Breathe in for five seconds. Then hold your breath for five seconds while tensing your entire body. Breathe out for five seconds as you relax your body. Repeat for three sets.

- To finish the routine, bring your focus back to your breathing and open your eyes when you feel ready.

- It is not uncommon to feel sleepy or even fall asleep during this, and for that reason, it can also be a great thing to do late at night when you go to bed, especially if you are struggling to sleep.

Relaxation is about switching off from your day and focusing on your breathing and your body, rather than what's going on in your head.

32 TOP TIPS FOR STAYING MOTIVATED

We are at the end of the book and in this list I'm not going to say anything radically new! That's because everything I have shared so far is based on a set of simple principles and not lots of complicated or unrealistic rules. The list below incorporates many of the themes I have repeated throughout the book, making it a one-stop shop so you can give yourself a quick pep talk when needed to help you stay on track with your plans to get healthier.

1 NEVER LOSE SIGHT OF YOUR GOAL

It might be a photo or a comment, not being able to play football with your kids or fit into clothes or worrying that you'll end up with type 2 diabetes like your father, but once this trigger point happens and you decide 'enough is enough', that's the start of a process that may take many months or even a year or more, and when the going gets tough, you will need to dig deep and push on through. At those times, remind yourself of what triggered your decision to change and the importance of your goal.

Of course, along the way, you will have many more goals. You will have daily and weekly goals. Love your goals. No matter how big or small, they will keep you on the right path.

2 DO IT TODAY!

If you have reached your 'enough is enough' moment, don't hesitate for another moment. Don't put it off or wait till Monday or 'till after the holidays'. There will always be something coming up. Make that commitment now, today, that you are going to make a change and do everything in your power to make it happen.

Write down three small goals you can achieve in the next 24 hours that will help to improve your health. Nothing crazy, just simple things you know you will be able to do. For instance, the first one could be to stop looking at screens 30 minutes before bedtime. You could do that tonight!

3 DON'T TELL PEOPLE ABOUT YOUR GOAL

As much as I admire people for posting and tweeting about what they are going to do, for most people, it just makes things harder! The more people you tell, the more pressure you are putting on yourself. When you fall off the wagon, as you will, it will be harder to get back on. Aim to do it for yourself. Tell those close to you and then just get on with it and make it happen. You don't owe anyone explanations for what you're eating or how you're exercising. If they comment on your choices, just brush it off pleasantly without getting into it. If someone who doesn't know that you are trying to get healthier says you look great, that will be all the recognition you need.

4 REMEMBER, RESULTS TAKE TIME!

Stop buying products or joining gyms/classes that promise unrealistic results. Results take time. Anyone who tells you differently is not telling the truth. Pick a goal that you can work towards over time – say,

Love your goals. No matter how big or small, they will keep you on the right path.

running a little further in the same time, losing 2lbs of weight – once you're moving towards the goal, you are getting there!

Take it one day at a time. Pick the simplest change that you can and build upon it a week at a time. Small changes add up to bigger changes over time and will be easier to do, as they won't seem as scary. There is so much content in this book that will improve your health; pick the tips that seem the most doable at the outset and go for it.

5 REACH FOR THE STARS!

Having advised you repeatedly to do things at your own pace, now I'm going to say something that will sound like a contradiction of that: think big! Be ambitious!

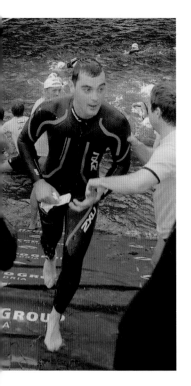

At some point, why not aim for something epic? Something that seems almost beyond you, but there is still a good chance that you will be able to do it if you prepare properly. All too often we settle for average when we are capable of so much more. For me, it was running a marathon, then doing an Ironman and then an ultramarathon – and that's despite not being a great runner. (The picture on the left is from when I competed in the Ironman in Austria ten years ago!)

6 ENJOY DOWNTIME

You should have at least one day a week when you rest and relax, doing no exercise or work and just unwinding. Doing this will help to reduce your stress levels and refresh your mind. Long-term health, real health, is about leading a balanced lifestyle.

7 GET BACK ON THE WAGON!

Remember, no one is perfect and change is hard. Chances are that you will fall off the wagon at some stage. You may do it a few times. Everybody does. The key is that you get back on track as soon as possible. You need to draw a line in the sand, accept that you have had a bad day/week and move forward. Beating yourself up and feeling guilty is only going to feed into a spiral of negative thoughts, which will be no good for your motivation. Simply give it no more thought.

8 LEARN TO CALM YOURSELF

Mindfulness has never been more popular, with lots of different versions and concepts. One of the simplest suggestions I can make is this: leave your phone at your desk when you go for lunch – you will be surprised at the calming effect this has on your lunch break!

Another simple way to meditate is to focus on your breathing. Breathe in through the nose for five seconds and then out through the mouth for five seconds. Breathe in as deeply as you can and try to get all the air out on the exhalation. Repeat this cycle ten times, thinking about nothing else but your breath.

Check out apps such as Calm, which will give you a structured meditation.

Remember, no one is perfect and change is hard.

9 BE GRATEFUL

Be thankful for what you have, not regretful for what you don't have. One of the issues with social media is that it is full of photographs of people showing off about how great their lives are – or appear to be. This can lead to envy and all the feelings that go with it. The reality is that you never know what's behind that photo. They are often designed to create the image of perfection, with filters and edits. No one's life is perfect, no matter how it seems online.

Having goals to aim for is brilliant, but never lose sight of the fact that what you have now is also good. Look around you and be thankful for all the great things you have in your life. At the end of the week, note down five things for which you are grateful from the past week – for example, the kind person who stopped to help you mend a puncture; the fact that you can easily afford good fresh food when so many people struggle; the project in work that got postponed when you were already snowed under; your granny's hip operation going so well; indeed, your granny (complete with gammy hips)… As you can see, the things that make you thankful don't have to be high-minded or complicated. Research into positive psychology shows that the act of thinking about and writing down things for which you are grateful has a powerful impact on your mindset and mood.

Having goals to aim for is brilliant, but never lose sight of the fact that what you have now is also good.

10 SURROUND YOURSELF WITH POSITIVITY

As much as possible, surround yourself with positivity, from friends to colleagues to mentors, as this will encourage you to be the best that you can be. As the saying goes, 'Fly with the eagles if you want to become an eagle yourself.'

This also applies to your health. We are normally the result of the people that we spend time with. If your friends spend the weekend in the pub and eat takeaways all week then the chances are that's what you are going to do too. I'm not saying that you should ditch your friends, but I am saying that you may need to find new ways of socializing with them and develop new networks as well – with people whose ideas about food and exercise are more aligned with your own. This will have an enormous influence on your health.

Here are the top five habits of people who live longer and live more healthily – hang out with folks like these and you'll be on the right path!

- They eat real foods and remove processed foods from their diets. They also tend to cook more, eating what would now be regarded as an old-school diet of staple foods.

- They are active on a daily basis, finding a form of exercise that they love.

- They see work as a pleasure rather than a chore. They get out of bed with a positive mindset in the morning, looking forward to taking on the day as opposed to dreading it.

- They don't sweat the small stuff. People who live longer have lower stress levels and an ability to step away from a stressful situation and make an informed decision.

- They are happier. Happier people are healthier, with lower resting heart rates and lower visceral fat levels. Happy people make better decisions in terms of food and exercise.

As much as possible, surround yourself with positivity, from friends to colleagues to mentors, as this will encourage you to be the best that you can be.

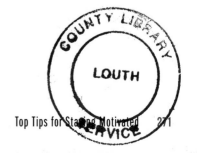
COUNTY LIBRARY
LOUTH
SERVICE

ACKNOWLEDGEMENTS

Acknowledgements are always so hard to write! In my life, I am lucky to be surrounded by wonderful people who support me all the way. They help me to achieve my goal of telling as many people as possible how to get healthier and fitter and to live more positive lives. Without them, I wouldn't have had the opportunity to write this book.

Hoping that I don't leave anyone out, here goes – big hugs and huge thanks to the following:

My agent Noel Kelly and the amazing Niamh T, Tara, Niamh M, Brian, Catriona and Jenny at NK Management.

Michael McLoughlin, Patricia Deevy and everyone at Penguin Ireland; the Raw Alchemy team – Paul McCarthy who took the photographs and Anne Kennedy who styled the recipe pictures; chef Aisling Boyle who worked with me on the recipes and on the shoot; my super neighbours, Natalie and Paul, who kindly demonstrated the exercises for the fitness section; and TJ from Columbia Sportswear for the support and help over the years.

Vision Independent Productions and RTÉ – for eleven years, and counting, working to get the nation healthier; and Independent Newspapers for giving me the chance to air my thoughts weekly.

My clients – you give me the most amazing sense of pride daily as I watch you change your lives.

My wonderful family who have always pushed me to believe that I can do anything.

My beautiful wife, whose never-ending patience and faith in all I try to do astounds me – love to you!

And finally, thanks to you – the reader – for buying this book. Thank you for taking a leap of faith and deciding to change your life. Believe in yourself and go for it!